MENDEL'S GARDEN:
SELECTED MEDICAL TOPICS

MENDEL'S GARDEN: SELECTED MEDICAL TOPICS

David J Holcombe

authorHOUSE®

AuthorHouse™ LLC
1663 Liberty Drive
Bloomington, IN 47403
www.authorhouse.com
Phone: 1-800-839-8640

Published by AuthorHouse   01/20/2014

ISBN: 978-1-4918-5021-3 (sc)
ISBN: 978-1-4918-5022-0 (e)

ACKNOWLEDGEMENTS
& DISCLAIMER

"MENDEL'S GARDEN: SELECTED MEDICAL TOPICS" is not intended to be a comprehensive text of current medical knowledge. It is a collection of selected texts of general interest, mostly published locally in "Visible Horizon" and "CENLA Focus." They do not represent official views of Dr. Holcombe's current or former employers, but simply the observations and opinions of the author. The title refers to the monk and great scientist, Gregor Mendel, who elucidated the principles of genetics while working in isolation and obscurity in his monastery in Moravia, perhaps not a little unlike Central Louisiana.

Most of the selections deal with subjects of general interest, although a few are more specialized and regional in nature. The order is somewhat arbitrary, with "Chronic Disease" starting the collection and "Lagniappe," ("a little extra" in Louisiana French) bringing up the rear. These texts do not contain all pertinent scientific references, although some useful references are cited from time to time for the benefit of the reader. This collection is destined to provide the non-scientific public with a place to start his or her explorations of the fascinating, but often confusing world of medicine.

Scientific texts are usually outdated as soon as (or even before) they are printed, and this publication will certainly not be exceptions to that rule. That is the inexorable march of medicine, and the sad fate of all scientific print publications. That being said, it is hoped that there is a consistent voice and perspective that will help situate these medical musings in the context of our unique set of social circumstances at this particular time in our social development. While diseases are more or less universal and often timeless, their frequency and the way they are treated vary from country to country, from social system to social system, and from one decade to the next. The result is an extraordinary diversity of medical outcomes (and costs) around the world depending on many complex factors.

As a reader, you may or may not agree with my personal perspectives on many medical issues, some of which are controversial. Fortunately, we live in a land where diversity of opinions is both encouraged and expected. As Puck implores in Shakespeare's *A Mid-Summer's Night Dream*, be not offended by these transient musings. Hopefully, you will pick up a few useful facts that may benefit you and your family and perhaps stimulate discussion with your friends and colleagues.

I would like to extend my sincere thanks to Terry Strickland, who painted my portrait on the cover, "Cranial Inspiration" in 2013.

David J. Holcombe, M.D., M.S.A., F.A.C.P.

January 2014

TABLE OF CONTENTS

CHAPTER I
CHRONIC DISEASES

CHAPTER II
CANCER

CHAPTER III
INFECTIOUS AND SEXUALLY TRANSMITTED DISEASES

CHAPTER IV
EAT, DRINK AND BE SICK

CHAPTER V
MEDICATIONS, DRUGS, TESTS AND MACHINES

CHAPTER VI
CREEPY CRAWLERS (AND FLYERS, TOO)

CHAPTER VII
GERIATRIC ISSUES

CHAPTER VIII
INFANTS, CHILDREN AND ADOLESCENTS

CHAPTER IX
HEALTHCARE
OUTCOMES AND POLICY

CHAPTER X
LAGNIAPPE (A LITTLE EXTRA)

CHAPTER I
CHRONIC DISEASES

A. CARDIOVASCULAR DISEASE

Despite significant reductions in heart attacks and strokes since the 1950's, cardiovascular disease (CVD) remains the leading cause of death in the United States. Every year 33.3% of deaths in men (398,563) and 35.3 % of deaths in women (432,709) are caused by CVD. Similar percentages are found in white and black populations, with slightly lower values among Hispanics.

Louisiana, with its high rates of obesity and smoking, ranks 46th out of 50 states for CVD deaths (308.4/100,000 population) and 46th for stroke deaths (52/100,000 population). Needless to say, the lower the rank, the bigger the problem it represents. There has been a reduction in death rates for CVD and stroke from 1996 to 2006 in Louisiana as well in the United States in general, but much work remains to be done.

The risk factors for CVD and stroke remain the same: hypertension, high cholesterol, obesity, diabetes, and, of course, tobacco use. There has been remarkable progress in the treatments for hypertension, diabetes and high cholesterol. At this time, a wide variety of excellent medications exist for treatment of all of these conditions. Also, smoking in the United States has decreased steadily over the last two decades, even though Louisiana still remains higher than the national average (22% vs. 19%) for smokers.

Much of the wonderful progress in the treatment of the risk factors for heart disease is being negated by the epidemic of obesity. Obesity, which now affects over 30% of the population of Louisiana, predisposes to diabetes, and diabetes (with or without hypertension) increases the risk for heart disease and stroke.

The sad fact about hypertension, high cholesterol and diabetes is that they can all be diagnosed by simple clinical or laboratory tests, yet they remain undiagnosed in a large segment of the population. About a quarter of diabetics are undiagnosed and untreated, and the same holds true for those with hypertension and high cholesterol. These three silent killers contribute to clogging of the arteries with atherosclerosis, which in turn leads to subsequent heart attacks and strokes.

Regular checks of blood pressure, cholesterol and blood sugars should be a normal part of ongoing medical surveillance. Everyone should have a primary care physician to assist them in the process of diagnosis and treatment. Ignorance is not bliss. And what you don't know might, in fact, kill you.

Although women live longer than men, more women die of heart disease than men. Their symptoms are often less obvious than those in men. Instead of classic arm and chest pain, women may only have unusual fatigue, shortness of breath, or vague digestive complaints. Both woman and men need to be aware of their risks of CVD and act accordingly. Lose weight, diagnosis and treat underlying risk factors, including hypertension, hypercholesterolemia, diabetes and smoking, and never ignore persistent symptoms, however typical they may seem. The life you save may be your own.

www.cdc.gov/heartdisease/index.htm

www.heart.org/HEARTORG/

http://www.cdc.gov/vitalsigns/heartdisease-stroke/index.html

B. HYPERTENSION: THE QUIET KILLER

Despite the presence of very effective medications, hypertension (high blood pressure) remains rampant. Nearly one in three Americans has high blood pressure (68 million). Of those with known hypertension, at least a third of those do not get treatment (20 million). Worse yet, of those who are being treated, around one half do not have adequate control of their blood pressure (37 million).

Hypertension is, indeed, a silent killer. Much like diabetes or elevated cholesterol, high blood pressure does not usually make people feel sick. Occasionally, when it is very high, people may have symptoms such as headaches or dizziness, but most of the time it asymptomatic (no symptoms at all). That does not, however, mean it is harmless. High blood pressure contributes directly to hardening of the arteries and a subsequent increased risk of heart disease and stroke. In fact, someone dies of heart attack, stroke or other cardiovascular disease every 39 seconds in the United States (over 800,000 deaths/year).

Medical treatment options have multiplied over the last decades and we now have a host of pharmaceutical treatment options including beta-blockers, Angiotensin Converting Enzyme (ACE) inhibitors, Angiotensin-Renin-Blockers (ARBs), centrally acting agents, various forms of diuretics and others. Some of these medications are available in generic forms that are safe, effective and inexpensive.

Before even trying medications, however, some simple measures should be employed, including weight reduction, reduced salt intake and smoking cessation. All three factors, obesity, salt and tobacco, act directly to aggravate hypertension and are contributing factors to the ravages of stroke and heart disease. Yet 30% of adult Louisiana residents remain obese and another 30% are overweight, making us one of the fattest states in the United States. Smoking rates in Louisiana also exceed the national averages (22% vs. 19%).

Although we should consume less than 2,000 milligrams of salt a day, many people consume two or three times that amount. Processed foods, even those "healthy low-fat diet foods" often contain huge amounts of salt to enhance taste. A can of soup or a few slices of pizza can contain over 1,000 milligrams of salt (half our recommended daily intake). Pickles, sauces, processed meats and almost all fast foods are loaded with salt, clearly indicated on food labels, largely in response to public tastes.

Paradoxically, most people (around 80%) with high blood pressure have access to health care. It is not simply a problem of decreased access to care, but a problem of inability or unwillingness to eat correctly, exercise adequately, take the medications that have been prescribed and stop smoking.

Every American should have their blood pressure checked regularly. Values greater than 140/90 should be rechecked, and, if verified, should result in life style changes and possibly medications. Those over 65 can have a systolic blood pressure up to 150, but above that is abnormal for them, too. Medications have never been so numerous or accessible, even to those with limited incomes, so treatment should never be delayed.

Cardiovascular diseases, the direct result of elevated blood pressure (and often associated cholesterol and diabetes) cost $300 billion dollars a year. This represents almost 20% of U.S. medical costs, which are already the highest in the world. Let us not just talk about reducing the national debt, but also about reducing the national waistline, salt intake, and epidemic high blood pressure. Don't be a statistic! Be part of the solution to this national health crisis, not part of the problem.

www.mayoclinic.com/health/high-blood-pressure/DS00100

http://www.cdc.gov/VitalSigns/CardiovascularDisease/index.html

http://www.cdc.gov/mmwr/preview/mmwrhtml/mm6004a4. htm?s_cid=mm6004a4_w

C. OBESITY, DIABETES AND HEALTHCARE

Obesity has reached epidemic proportions. One third of all adults in Louisiana have a BMI (Body Mass Index) of 30 or greater, putting them in the obese category. Sixty percent of all Louisianans are either overweight or obese. Even more alarming, around 20% of children in our state from 10 to 17 are also obese, an increase of several percentage points since 2003. Louisianans share this sad privilege with the other states in the lower Mississippi River area, as well as those in Coastal Carolina and Appalachian counties.

This gradual increase in obesity has been creeping across the United States over the last few decades, just as levels of physical activity have declined in a significant proportion of the population. This has been especially true among children, only 25% of whom meet the recommendations for physical activity in high school. While activity has dwindled, screen time among children has increased. In Louisiana, one third of all high school students watch over three hours of television a day and over 70% have a TV in their bedrooms, something that directly increases the risk of childhood obesity.

These dismal statistics, especially among children, bode ill for the future. Obesity is directly related to the subsequent development of diabetes, hypertension and heart disease, all of them life-threatening conditions. The combination of diabetes and hypertension results in huge increases in strokes in both black and white populations. Add to this our higher than national averages of tobacco use in Louisiana (and the South in general), and you have a perfect storm of medical misery.

As weights have ballooned, so have the associated medical problems and their associated costs. Diabetes, directly associated to increases in weight, also results in increases in renal failure, blindness, and peripheral vascular disease and associated amputations. Yet our collective weights continue to increase as if there were no consequences to our actions.

Why has this obesity epidemic become such an important issue? First, it poses a huge health risk to those who suffer from it. Diabetes is a silent, long-term killer that increases disability as it shortens lives. Second, obesity, and subsequent diabetes, also poses a risk to the entire healthcare system. The phenomenal expense associated with diabetic medications, dialysis, surgical corrections of peripheral and cardiac disease, rehabilitation from stokes and heart attacks and the associated loss of productivity run in the billions. Much of this cost is avoidable. We are not compelled to eat ourselves into personal and collective calamity.

Everyone, especially in Louisiana, enjoys the pleasure associated with good food and fellowship. We must never forget, however, that the hidden costs of obesity include the loss of both health and prosperity. An ounce of prevention will prevent a pound of cure. Those who lament the future bankruptcy of their children and children's children should understand that our efforts to stem the current epidemic of obesity will help prevent such an avoidable economic catastrophe.

Prevention, once again, is the key. Although there have been wonderful, dramatic improvements in the treatment of diabetic related conditions, the secret remains avoiding diabetes in the first place. Reduce your calorie intake, increase your physical activity, and, if you have the misfortune of already suffering from diabetes, do everything in your power to maintain it under control. Adequate diabetic control, while not a 100% guarantee of avoiding complications, greatly reduces them in the long run. It is up to us as individuals, and collectively as a society, to address obesity and reduce its terrible burden in personal suffering and medical costs. Your doctor is your best ally in this fight, but he or she cannot win this battle without the full cooperation of the patient.

www.mayoclinic.com/health/obesity/DS00314

www.cdc.gov/obesity/

http://obesityinamerica.org/

D. SMOKE AND MIRRORS:
THE DEADLY ILLUSION

Tobacco kills. As glamorous and harmless as the tobacco industry tries to make it, smoking contributes to 40% of all deaths (over 450,000) in the U.S. every year. It surpasses the negative effects of poor diet and physical inactivity, which "only" contribute to 35% of all deaths.

The slaughter from tobacco takes the form of lung cancer (29%), heart disease (28%), chronic lung disease (21%), other cancers (8%), strokes (4%) and a smattering of other illnesses. Besides death, smoking (whether first hand or second hand) also contributes to bone loss (osteoporosis), pre-mature menopause, decreased vision and hearing and wrinkles.

Smoking is particularly devastating to women, contributing to delays in conception, increased spontaneous abortions and stillbirths, lower birth weights, and higher risks for Sudden Infant Death Syndrome (SIDS) and cognitive deficits in newborns. In fact, smoking more than doubles the risk for low birth weights and children born with serious medical conditions.

Despite this deluge of information, around 20% of Americans still smoke (22.2% of men and 17.4% of women.) These rates can be as high as 25% in Central Louisiana. Smoking rates are inversely proportional to education and income, with more well-to-do and educated people smoking less. Since Central Louisiana has low per capita income ($26,000 vs. $46,000 nationally) and fewer college graduates (10% vs. 24% nationally), it is not surprising we have higher than national smoking rates. It is an explanation, but not an excuse.

As mentioned above, women tend to pay a higher health cost than men. A woman's risk for heart disease and heart attacks are double that of man, while she is 13 times more likely to develop emphysema or lung cancer.

Even though smoking rates have decreased in the United States, smokers still consume 18.6 billion packs annually, with an average price of $4.80 per pack. Taxes vary from state to state, with an average of $1.31 (only 36 cents/pack in Louisiana). Yet despite the tax revenues, health care costs per pack run from $8.37 to $10.40 or 96 billion dollars in direct medical costs and 97 billion in indirect costs (lost time and disability).

While women were latecomers to the tobacco habit, they have been the subjects of intense marketing pressure by cigarette makers. There has been a concerted effort to make smoking look glamorous and sexy. Packaging and publicity are often directed specifically at women, as well as minorities and adolescents, in the hopes of ensnaring new, susceptible populations. Almost all regular smokers in the U.S. started smoking prior to 18 years of age, a fact well known to the tobacco industry. With increased restriction in the United States, tobacco marketing has shifted to overseas markets, also targeting women and young people. Tobacco, just like money, never sleeps.

We should seek every opportunity and every means to reduce tobacco use. While smoking injures the user, it also attacks unborn children, living children and all those who are subjected to second hand smoke. Let us do everything in our power to eliminate the unnecessary health and economic burdens inflicted by tobacco. If you smoke, stop. If you do not, seek ways to decrease this unnecessary burden on our society. Let's clear the air!

www.cdc.gov/tobacco/data_statistics/fact_sheets/health_effects/tobacco_related_mortality/

E. CELEBRATING THE ALEXANDRIA SMOKE-FREE ORDINANCE

On October 4, 2011, the Alexandria City Council unanimously passed the Local Smoke-Free Ordinance, legislation that removed the state exemption for standalone bars, gaming facilities, tobacco shops, and certain rooms in nursing homes. The ordinance also requires smokers to remain at least 25 feet from an entrance to any building. The city ordinance compliments and strengthens provisions of the Louisiana Smoke-Free Air Act of 2006.

Why celebrate? First, Alexandria is the first city in Louisiana to pass such a progressive and comprehensive ordinance. Second, air quality readings verified the tremendous improvement in indoor air quality as a result of the ordinance, thus protecting countless lives. And third, economic impact appears to be minimal on targeted locations, although this is anecdotal and still under local study.

Why is this still an important issue? First, smoking remains a problem in Louisiana and the United States in general. Almost one in five Americans still smokes and over one in four Louisianans still smoke. Smoking remains the single largest contributing factor to emphysema and lung cancer, both costly and potentially avoidable problems. Over 50% of those who continue to smoke will go on to die from smoking-related problems. Smoking related deaths cost $96 billion each year in direct medical costs and the same in losses due to premature deaths.

Despite expenditures of almost 10 billion dollars a year on direct advertising by the tobacco industry, the number of Americans that smoke has decreased from 20.9% in 2005 to 19.3% in 2010. The percentage of heavy smokers (30/day or more) has decreased from 13% in 2005 to only 8% in 2010. In states with aggressive anti-smoking programs, such as California, the number of adults smoking has dropped by nearly 50% and the number of cigarettes smoked per person has plummeted by 67% since implementation of their initiatives in 1988.

Increased knowledge about the disastrous effects of smoking, more restrictive legislation about where smoking can occur, and increased cost of a pack of cigarettes, have all contributed to reduced cigarette use. The poor, minorities, women and youth, however, still remain targets of aggressive and insidious advertising. Among school children in Louisiana, 14.5% have smoked a cigarette prior to age 13 and 21.8% currently smoke (13% smoking over 10 cigarettes a day). Everyone, especially tobacco companies, recognize that if a young person less than 21 years of age starts smoking, he or she will remain a smoker for the rest of their shortened lives.

We need to celebrate every action at a local, state and national level that promotes health by restricting tobacco, one of the most dangerous products legally available. You cannot make people lead healthy lives, but you can protect those who have no choice (those exposed to second hand smoke) and you can reduce the opportunities for self-destruction by those who choose to indulge.

Congratulations Alexandria for your comprehensive Smoke Free Ordinance! It is hoped that similar ordinances will appear in other Louisiana cities and parishes. This is a winnable battle to reduce the ravages of preventable illness. Both public awareness and public policies together are needed to overcome personal misinformation and aggressive misleading marketing.

F. FIBROMYALGIA: PROBLEM AND OPPORTUNITY

Fibromyalgia has evolved over the last few decades from a hypothesis to a recognized entity by the American College of Rheumatology. Despite the extensive press and popular support that surrounds this disease entity, there remains a fair amount of skepticism in the medical community about what this disease represents and how best to treat it.

The generally accepted view is that fibromyalgia represents a disorder of pain reception and transfer. Starting with physical and psychological stressors, the sufferer's body somehow amplifies the pain signals, resulting in an increased perception of pain. Studies seem to show that certain areas of the brain are differentially affected, resulting in long term effects, up to and including decrease in brain volume.

Some people seem to have a genetic pre-disposition related to their metabolism of the neurotransmitters serotonin and dopamine, endorphins, as well as in the interleukin-1 immune response. No single gene appears to play a predominant role and fibromyalgia is not, strictly speaking, a genetic disease. Some experts call it the quintessential mind-body disorder, which affects nerves, the endocrine and immune systems as well as the psychological wellbeing of the patient.

Sufferers may display a constellation of symptoms besides pain, which may include fatigue, depression, memory loss, insomnia, loss of concentration, and a propensity to suffer from irritable bowel syndrome. It is estimated that 2 to 5% of people worldwide suffer from fibromyalgia and that it strikes women, predominantly between 35 to 60 years of age, ten times more often than men. It can affect younger women as well, especially if there has been a history of psychological or sexual abuse in childhood.

For a diagnosis, the American College of Rheumatology requires that the patient have symptoms lasting over three months and that there be at least 11/18 positive trigger points (specific areas of the body that are painful to palpation.) Fibromyalgia is not the same as "chronic widespread pain syndrome" since 15-25% of those individuals do not meet the criteria for fibromyalgia.

Treatment includes non-pharmacological modalities such as exercise and psychological therapy. Medications, approved by the FDA, include Pregabalin (*Lyrica*), Duloxetine (*Cymbalta*) and Milnacipran (*Savella*). These agents, sometimes used together, can have significant side effects. In addition, they are extremely expensive. Curiously, the United States is the only country that officially approves of these medications for use in fibromyalgia.

Because of the non-specific nature of many of the complaints and the fact that there is no blood or radiological test to confirm the diagnosis of fibromyalgia, it still elicits a fair amount of skepticism in significant segments of the medical community. Although it has been said that there is "no role for therapeutic Nihilism in the treatment of fibromyalgia," the complexity and cost of the treatment discourages many providers, since behavioral aspects must be addressed as well as somatic ones. Solid scientific research as well the development of more cost effective treatments would do much to help relieve the enormous numbers of people who suffer from some manifestations of this mysterious and occasionally debilitating disorder.

www.cdc.gov/arthritis/basics/fibromyalgia.htm

G. ARTHRITIS: PROGRESS AND PROBLEMS

Arthritis continues to be a major medical issue in the United States and elsewhere. A study in 2007 revealed that the number of Americans with some form of arthritis increased from 36.8 million in 1997 to 46.1 million in 2003. It is estimated that this number will reach 67 million in 2030, fueled by the tidal wave of aging Baby Boomers. During the same period from 1997 to 2003, the cost of treating arthritis rose from $88 billion to $322 billion a year (or about 1 percent of the gross domestic product of the United States) and will probably double by 2013.

While there are many forms of arthritis, osteoarthritis or degenerative joint disease alone affects over 21 million people in the United States and results in 7 million doctor visits a year. Rheumatoid arthritis, a progressive crippling arthritic variant affects over 2 million Americans, often striking in middle age and affecting twice as many women as men. While the numbers are staggering, there have been remarkable advances in medical care, especially for rheumatoid arthritis.

Since rheumatoid arthritis involves immunologically modulated destruction of joints, there has been a proliferation of agents that specifically modify this self-destructive process. These so-called "biologics" include Tissue Necrosis Factor Alpha inhibitors such as etanercept (*Enbrel*), infliximab (*Remicade*), adalimumab (*Humera*), golimumab (*Simponi*) and cerolozumab (*Cimizia*). These "miracle drugs," as well as other immumnomodulators such as anakinra (*Kineret*), abatacept (*Orencia*), rituximab (*Rituxan*) and tocilizumab (*Actemra*) have transformed the evolution of rheumatoid arthritis by interrupting the destruction and allowing long-term remissions, thus avoiding crippling deformations.

Such "miracle drugs," however, come with elevated price tags and have multiplied the cost of treatment when compared with certain older, generic medications such as methotrexate. As Dr. Donnellan commented "The price of new products to treat rheumatoid arthritis represents a huge leap in the cost of treatment. However, the improvements in treatment offered by these drugs are driving their use in spite of the high cost." To compound the problem, earlier diagnosis and longer periods of treatment only add to the overall costs, which can exceed $2,000 a month. Direct-to-consumer (DTC) advertising also increased demand, despite formulary restrictions that may exist.

It is estimated that more than 40% of all rheumatoid patients have problems with the cost of their treatment, and almost 40% of this group cannot afford the more expensive "biologics." Factors related to cost have slowed the acceptance of these drugs in Europe, where use is about a fourth of that in the U.S. despite an equal or greater number of sufferers. Many patients in the U.S. are left with the unsavory choice of forgoing treatment, or accepting treatments with less chance of delaying disease-related withdrawal from the workforce, something which occurs in 50% of newly diagnosed cases within ten years.

For those who need medication assistance, several companies offer Patient-Assistance Programs (PAPs). These include Abbott, Bristol-Myers Squibb, Pfizer, Janssen and others. The paperwork involved can be cumbersome and poses an impediment to their use in some cases, sometimes derisively called "rationing by inconvenience."

At least in Louisiana, the Rapides Foundation sponsors C-MAP, a medical assistance program with a statewide presence. Community Health Worx, a free working people's clinic in Alexandria, also provides medication assistance to those without insurance. There are also national organizations such as NeedyMeds.org and The HealthWell Foundation that can help. As with many aspects of medical care in the United States and elsewhere, the questions becomes not what we have to offer medically, but what society in general and patients in particular can really afford.

http://www.cdc.gov/arthritis/basics/rheumatoid.htm

H. TO SCREEN OR NOT TO SCREEN, THAT IS THE QUESTION

Shakespeare's Prince Hamlet asked the famous questions, "To be or not to be?" We can apply a variant of the questions to the subject of medical screenings, "To screen or not to screen?" At first glance, it would appear obvious that medical screenings are an absolute good, the more the better. Yet the reality is much more complicated and subtle. In fact, some screening tests are very good, some are questionable, and some do more harm than good. Why is this so?

Screening tests are designed to uncover specific diagnoses, whether they are colon cancer, breast cancer, aortic aneurisms, peripheral or carotid artery disease, hypertension, thyroid abnormalities, prostate cancer or many other conditions. No test is perfect, and each one can be evaluated based on how many cases of a particular condition can be successfully diagnosed in a given population. The cost and complexity of the test must also be factored in. There are a host of technical statistical terms related to evaluating testing such as true positives, false positives, positive and negative predictive value and other mathematical ways of evaluating the efficiency of a screening test.

The bottom line is how successful any test is in diagnosing a medical problem, and, of course, if the problem exists, will that diagnosis result in a subsequent treatment that will improve the quality and quantity of the patient's life at a reasonable cost?

The problem with testing for multiple conditions is that there are hundreds of possible screening tests, from simple and cheap determinations of blood pressure, to highly complex and expensive tests, such as colonoscopies, treadmill tests and CAT scans. While a test may be useful, it may be too expensive to perform on the general population or may result in a host of incorrect (false positive) diagnoses that, in turn, result in unnecessary, costly or even dangerous procedures.

So what is the answer? Should we not test at all in the hopes that ignorance is bliss, or should we undergo every available test, while running the risk of false positive exams, with subsequent expensive, nerve wracking and possibly dangerous work-ups?

In fact, the U.S. Preventative Services Task Force (USPSTF) already evaluates each test. The Task Force is comprised of independent experts who classify tests according to their benefit to the population. Each test receives a grade: A, B, C, D or I, depending upon the recommendations of the experts.

A: Recommend (High certainty the net benefit is substantial): Offer test.

B: Recommend (High certainty that net benefit is moderate): Offer test.

C: Do Not Provide Routinely (Consider for certain individual patients; moderate certainty that the net benefit is probably small).

D: Discourage the Use of This Service (No net benefit; harm outweighs benefit)

I: Insufficient Evidence for Recommendation

The U.S. Preventative Services Task Force strives to take some of the guesswork out of the complex decision-making surrounding screening tests for the doctors as well as the general public. Tests, which have received an "A" classification, include:

Lipid profile for men over 35 and women over 45

Biennial (every other year) **screening mammography** for women 50 to 74 years old

PAP smears for all sexually active women under 65 years of age

Colorectal screening for all people 50-75 years of age

HIV Testing for all high-risk adolescents and adults

There are others tests that are recommended in specific populations (such as aortic aneurism screening with ultrasound or blood pressure testing in asymptomatic adults.) It is easy to go to <u>www.uspreventiveservicestaskforce.org</u> and look up an individual test in multiple diagnostic categories.

An appropriate screening test may save your life. An inappropriate test may put you through expensive, unnecessary further testing and emotional turmoil. Take the time to see which tests are really recommended. We already have the most expensive medical delivery system in the world. Let's make it more efficient by relying on verifiable medical evidence. Screen when it's appropriate, pass when it's not. Can we answer our questions "To test or not to test?" Well, as with many things in life, it just depends.

<u>www.uspreventiveservicestaskforce.org</u>

CHAPTER II
CANCER

A. COLON AND RECTAL CANCER AWARENESS

There are over 100,000 new cases of colon cancer diagnosed in the United States each year and almost 50,000 deaths. Around 1,000 Louisiana's will die each year from this preventable disease. Louisiana has higher rates than the national averages in incidences (new cases) of colorectal cancer for men (71.3 LA vs. 61.3 U.S.) and women (48.9 LA vs. 42.1 U.S.) It also has higher rates for deaths from colorectal cancer for men (29.2 LA vs. 24.4 US) and women (18.8 LA vs. 15.4 U.S.) In other words, more Louisianans get colorectal cancer and more of them die from it than the national averages. Both incidences and death rates are significantly higher in blacks than whites.

Most, if not all, of these colo-rectal cancer deaths are preventable. Early diagnosis leads to far better results: 89.8% five year survival for localized cancer versus 67.7% survival for regional cases and only 10.3% five year survival for cases with distant disease (metastases) at diagnosis. With better awareness and systematic use of colonoscopy for those 50 years and above, 5 year survival rates have increased from 51% (in 1975-77) to over 65% (in 1996-2003) for all stages combined.

Increasing the use of fecal occult blood testing (at the very least), or preferably colonoscopy in those 50 and above has been a constant goal of the medical community. The message, however, has not been equally received by all segments of the population. Insured non-Hispanic whites (with a high school education or less) are more likely to have received screening of any kind than insured blacks or Hispanics. The rates of screening for all racial groups drop by about half among the uninsured. The higher the educational level, the more likely any group was to have received screening.

Since screening establishes the extent of colorectal cancer at diagnosis, and stage at diagnosis determines survival, the earlier the diagnosis, the better the survival results. Unfortunately, survival is also related to insurance status. Insured patients do much better for all earlier stages of colorectal cancer than those with Medicaid or the uninsured, whose survival curves are virtually the same. Patients with advanced metastatic disease do poorly regardless of insurance status.

Every individual 50 years old and over, insured or not, should be aware of the importance of screening for colorectal cancer. If you have insurance, make sure that your physician offers at least fecal occult blood testing, or preferably a colonoscopy, when appropriate. For the 20% of the Louisiana population that benefits from Medicaid or the nearly 20% with no insurance at all, you must insist on periodic screening wherever you receive health care. If and when opportunities arise to undergo free screenings, they should be seized. No one enjoys the inconvenience and indignities of sampling stools or undergoing colonoscopy prep, but that inconvenience is nothing compared with the tragedy of an avoidable death from colorectal cancer.

www.cancer.gov/cancertopics/types/colon-and-rectal

www.mayoclinic.com/health/colon-cancer/DS00035

http://www.cdc.gov/cancer/colorectal/

B. BREAST CANCER: PROGRESS
AND OPPORTUNITIES

Although some progress has been made, breast cancer remains the most frequently diagnosed cancer among woman in the United States (29%) and Louisiana (26%). Over 13,000 women die each year of breast cancer in the U.S. (around 750 of them in Louisiana alone.) Almost 3,000 women are diagnosed with new breast cancer each year.

Women have understood that clinical breast exams, begun after age 20, and screening mammograms, begun at age 40 (or earlier with a positive family history), help to improve outcomes through earlier diagnosis. This has resulted in declining mortality rates from breast cancer in the United States as a whole. In fact, five-year survival rates have increased from 75% (1975-77) to 89% (1996-2003), a 14% increase. The facts are clear: the earlier the diagnosis, the better the outcome, with survivals increasing dramatically with an earlier stage at diagnosis.

The situation becomes much more complex when race and insurance status are introduced. Insured white women are more likely to be diagnosed in Stage I (an earlier stage) than uninsured white women. And both insured and uninsured black and Hispanic women are more likely to be diagnosed in Stage II, with correspondingly worse outcomes. In fact, survival for breast cancer is much worse in the uninsured and Medicaid patients than in those with insurance at any stage of diagnosis.

In Louisiana, the situation is the same or worse as nationally. Mortality rates among black women have actually been increasing in Louisiana, unlike in the United States in general (Louisiana Tumor Registry). Since mortality is directly related to stage at diagnosis, and mammograms help to increase the diagnosis of earlier cancers, then there must be a problem with early access to this procedure in Louisiana.

In fact, in Louisiana, like elsewhere in the United States, the percentage of women who get a mammogram is directly correlated with race, insurance status, and educational level. Insured women of any race get more mammograms than those who are uninsured, whether they be white, black, or Hispanic. Only around 20% of uninsured blacks or whites have gotten a mammogram in the last year, while this jumps to over 50% among the insured of any race. Central Louisiana has among the lowest rates of screening mammograms in the state.

Louisiana has particularly high numbers of uninsured (around 20%) and Medicaid recipients (25%), the very groups that are the least likely to get a mammogram and, once diagnosed, do the worst in survival. It is not surprising that our breast cancer mortality rates in Louisiana are higher than the national average (29.8 vs. 25.5) and that there is a marked black/white disparity within this group (40.9 vs. 25.3).

Women who undergo regular mammograms (with monthly self-exams) should continue to do so. Mammograms, while not foolproof, offer the best opportunity of early diagnosis, treatment, and possible cure. Women who do not undergo mammograms should be encouraged to do so. All barriers to this life-saving procedure should be reduced or eliminated. The social, emotional, and monetary costs of breast cancer treatment can be overwhelming. Let us reduce that burden by early diagnosis and treatment of as many women as possible, whatever the means.

www.cancer.gov/cancertopics/types/breast

www.cancer.org/cancer/breastcancer/

http://www.cdc.gov/cancer/breast/

C. IS FIFTY THE NEW FORTY?
WHEN TO GET A MAMMOGRAM

There has been a lot of controversy over the recommendations by the United States Preventative Services Task Force (USPSTF) for initiation of screening mammograms (not diagnostic mammograms related to abnormal clinical findings) beginning at age 50. This is in contradiction with the recommendations from the American Cancer Society for mammograms beginning at 40. This difference of opinions created quite a firestorm of protests, especially from breast cancer survivors under the age of 50 and their supporters, who passionately support the use of earlier mammograms.

How did we get to such a dilemma? How could two highly respected organizations come up with recommendations that differ by a decade?

Everyone recognizes the importance of mammograms. Breast cancer claimed 40,000 women in 2009. While still a high figure, deaths from breast cancer have decreased 2.3% per year during the 90's for all women and 3.3% per year for women between 40 and 50 years of age. No one denies the importance of mammograms in the early diagnosis of breast cancer, but there is question about the optimum time to begin.

The origin of the controversy resides in risk-benefit ratios. How many tests have to be done on how many women to make a test useful? In addition, what harm comes from doing the test? Since no test is 100% accurate, there will always be a number of false positive tests, leading to unnecessary, painful and costly further testing. There will also be a certain number of false negative, resulting in delays of diagnosis and worse outcomes. Both the American Cancer Society and the U.S. Preventative Services Task Force (USPSTF) examined the facts and came up with different conclusions.

The USPSTF decided that screening in women 40-49 should have a grade of C (meaning it did not qualify for medical coverage based on current evidence). For women 50 to 74 years of age, mammograms were given a grade of B (thus qualifying them for coverage). Mammograms for women 75 and above were not recommended.

How did they reach this conclusion? In fact, to save one woman's life (between the ages of 40-49), you have to do 1,900 mammograms. That number of mammograms will result in 1,330 callbacks, 665 breast biopsies, 8 diagnoses of cancer, and only one life saved. The number of mammograms necessary to save one life drops to 1,340 for women 50-59 and only 370 for women 60 to 69.

For a woman in her 40's the chance of being diagnosed with breast cancer is only 0.42%. But because of the large numbers of women being tested, that still translates into 11,751 avoidable deaths. For women in their fifties, that number increases to 15,330 avoidable deaths and rises to 37,592 for women in their 60's.

When sophisticated computer models are used, the most efficient interval for mammogram appears to be one every two years. As for starting dates, it remains a function of the goal being sought. It is 50 years old if the goal is the most efficient manner to reduce mortality and 40 years old if the goal is the maximization of years of life saved.

When the dust settled, recommendation of the American Cancer Society (ACS) remained in place. They still recommend annual mammograms starting at 40 years of age, with no stop date. Monthly self-exams are still recommended between 20-39 years of age, while recognizing that they offered no documented protective effect.

As with all imperfect tests, it is always a question of risk-benefit ratios. Because the cost of health care must become a limiting factor at some point, cost-benefit ratios will also have to be considered. There will always be a point where limited resources and unlimited demand collide. Asking the painful question of how much we can spend to save a life will, of necessity, have to be considered as unpleasant as that prospect may be.

www.cancer.gov/cancertopics/factsheet/detection/mammograms

http://www.cdc.gov/cancer/nbccedp/

D. PROSTATE CANCER:
TO TEST OR NOT TO TEST?

Prostate cancer remains the most diagnosed cancer in American men today (25% of all newly diagnosed cancers), followed by lung cancers at 15%. But while prostate cancer is the most common male cancer, it is a distant second to lung cancer as a cause of death (9% vs. 30%). At first glance, this may seem strange, yet it is related to the frequency and severity (or indolence) of prostate cancer. In fact, while lung cancer has an incidence to mortality ratio of 1.4 to 1, prostate cancer is only 7.1 to 1 or five times less deadly.

Autopsies performed on men, regardless of the cause of death, show that over 50% of men over fifty have evidence of prostate cancer, but only 18% are aware of their disease, and only 2% of them died from prostate cancer. After 70 years of age, 64% of men will have biopsy proven prostate cancer, regardless of their cause of death. Blacks are more prone to have this problem than whites and Asians are less likely. Anyone with a family history has an increased risk, which rises with age in all men. In short, there is a lot of prostate cancer out there, more in some groups than others, but most men will not die from it.

That being said, there exists excellent ways to diagnosis this common problem. A digital rectal exam is done in conjunction with a Prostate Specific Antigen (or PSA), a simple blood test. PSA is a substance secreted from the prostate and detectable in the blood. It rises in cases of prostate cancer, but also with inflammation of the prostate (prostatitis), a benign infectious disease. The introduction of the PSA around 1985 led to a huge increase in the diagnosis of cases, peaking around 1992. Suspecting cancer, however, is not the same as proving it. That requires a prostate biopsy (the insertion of a tube in the rectum and the removal of multiple cores of prostate tissue.) Those samples receive a histological grade, a Gleason Score (ranging from 2-10) or severity index of sorts, with more benign forms having a lower score than more aggressively malignant forms.

Early screening with annual PSA tests does reduce the risk of death by 25%. Yet it also almost doubles the chances of being diagnosed with prostate cancer, including a large number of cases with low Gleason Scores. Treatment for prostate cancer can include prostatectomy (removal of the prostate), which may result in a certain number of men with impotence (loss of sexual activity) and urinary incontinence, both very troubling side effects. Since older men have a significant chance of dying with prostate cancer and not from it, prostatectomy is recommended for those with higher Gleason Scores (6 and above) in patients younger than 65. There are, of course, lots of individual variations related to the stage, Gleason score and PSA values, which need to be discussed with your physician.

While understanding the complexity of the situation, the recommendation still remains (at least in the U.S.) to begin annual PSA testing at 50. Race, family history and age all play a role, with African-Americans being at higher risk and often starting testing at 45. The decision to be tested and the age at which testing should begin, as well as decisions about treatment, should be individualized, taking into consideration all the risks and benefits of treatment versus watchful waiting. Whatever the decision, it should be an informed one after a discussion with your primary care physician or urologist.

www.cdc.gov/cancer/prostate/basic_info/screening.htm

http://www.mayoclinic.com/health/prostate-cancer/HQ01273

E. SUN EXPOSURE:
TOO MUCH OF A GOOD THING

Most people love the sun, but as with many things, too much of a good thing causes serious problems. Limited exposure to sunlight is actually beneficial and results in the activation of Vitamin D, essential for the formation of healthy bones. Inadequate levels of Vitamin D secondary to low dietary intake or little or no sun exposure, can lead to osteomalacia or rickets, a rare disorders resulting in soft bones.

Our most common health problem, however, is not too little sun exposure, but too much. Ultraviolet rays result in destructive changes in skin that decrease elastic tissue (causing wrinkles) and, more importantly, cause alterations in skin cells that cause skin cancer. Skin cancers are the most common form of cancer, with over 3.5 million cases diagnosed each year in the United States. New cases of skin cancer exceed the number of new cases of breast, prostate and colon cancers combined. One in five Americans will be diagnosed with skin cancer in their lifetime and 50% of those aged 50-65 will develop a skin cancer.

Sun exposure increases the risk of all forms of skin cancers: basocellular carcinomas, squamous cell carcinomas and melanomas. Basocellular carcinomas, the most common form of skin cancers, are frequently found on the sun-exposed areas, particularly the tip of the nose, the ears, and the back of the hands. Although usually superficial and less deadly than other forms of skin cancer, basocellulars often require surgical removal, which can leave unsightly scarring. Squamous cell carcinomas are more aggressive and can metastasize to regional lymph nodes, resulting in the need for extensive surgery and radiation. Even with proper treatment, squamous cell carcinomas cause over 2,500 deaths a year.

Although melanomas represent less than 5% of skin cancers, they cause 75% of all skin cancer deaths. One in 55 people will develop a melanoma and it is the most common cancer in those aged 25-29. When diagnosed early, survival rates exceed 99%, but fall to 15% or less in more advanced stages. Since almost all melanomas are caused by ultraviolet radiation, the rate of new melanomas has risen by 45% between 1992 and 2004 with increased outdoor activities (and tanning). Over 120,000 new cases were diagnosed in 2011 and 8,790 people died from melanomas that same year. Every mole that appears to be enlarging, bleeding, itching, becoming irregular and darkening should be considered suspect and removed.

Sun exposure is the common culprit for all skin cancers. Even one blistering sun burn in childhood doubles the risk of developing a melanoma, as does five or more sun burns by any age. Regular use of tanning parlors also increases the risk of melanoma by 75%. Frequent users are 2.5 times more likely to develop a squamous cell carcinoma and 1.5% more likely to develop a basocellular carcinoma. Clearly the risks of cancer exceed the dubious benefits of a tan.

Ultraviolet exposure from sun (or tanning) results in accumulated risk and the longer the lifetime exposure to sun, the greater the risk of developing skin cancer. Besides disfiguration and death, the economic cost of non-melanoma skin cancers (basocellular and squamous cell carcinomas) exceeds 1.5 billion a year, while the cost of melanoma treatment alone approaches $250 million.

The bottom line is that excessive sun exposure is bad for you. Use hats, gloves and long sleeve shirts when possible and always use sunscreen. Sunscreens should be able to block both ultraviolet B and A radiation. Ingredients vary, but whatever they are, they must offer a Sun Protection Factor (SPF) of at least 15 or greater. Water resistant broad-spectrum sun screens with a SPF of 30 or greater are recommended, especially for children.

Enjoy the outdoors, but protect yourself and your loved ones from the most common and most preventable of cancers, skin cancers.

www.skincancer.org

http://www.cdc.gov/cancer/skin/

F. THE COST OF CANCER CARE

A diagnosis of cancer strikes fear into the heart of most ordinary citizens. More than 1.5 million Americans were diagnosed with some form of cancer in 2010, 21,000 of them living in Louisiana. Although there are many different types of cancers, with many different prognoses, over 569,000 Americans died from cancer in 2010 (8,480 of them in Louisiana). The five most common cancers diagnosed in men in Louisiana from 2002-2006 were prostate (30%), lung (18%), colorectal (11%), bladder (6%) and kidney (4%). Among women, the most common cancers were breast (29%), lung (15%), colorectal (12%), uterine (4%) and non-Hodgkin lymphoma (4%).

Dying from cancer is always a possibility and that, is a fearful prospect. Compounding that fear is the growing issue of the economic cost of cancer care. No one suffering from any form or cancer wants to be burdened by the cost of treatment, but that cost of treatment has steadily risen with advances in technology and pharmacology. The cost of drugs related to cancer care has increased from $5 billion in 1998 to $19.2 billion in 2008. During this same time, the total cost of cancer care reached $104 billion in 2006 and promises to nearly double by 2020. The vast majority of new cancer drugs, approved within the last four years by the FDA, have exceeded $20,000 for a three-month treatment, which may prolong life by a scant 2 months or less. The cost of most new anti-cancer drugs exceeds $5,000 per month.

As Dr. Antonio Fojo of the National Cancer Institute stated in an American Society of Clinical Oncology interview, "When you charge $80,000 for a drug that gives a patient an average of 1.2 months survival advantage that just doesn't make sense. So we're giving these drugs to too many patients, including many patients who experience no benefit, and we are in fact causing them harm."

It has been shown that 20% of families will exhaust their savings while paying for medications involved with cancer care. Not only are families threatened, but the enormous increases in the cost of cancer contribute to the ballooning cost of medical care in general, now reaching over 2.7 trillion dollars a year (over $8,000/per capita/

year), or about 17% of the U.S. gross national product. That cost of all medical care is estimated to reach $4 trillion or more by 2015, or 20% of the gross national product, although it appears that costs may be leveling off somewhat around 18%.

What are the solutions for this dramatic situation? Can we afford to treat all patients under all circumstances, regardless of the cost? What can physicians do to reduce cost while still providing the compassionate care expected of all doctors. A recent article in the New England Journal of Medicine by Drs. Smith and Millner suggested a few changes. First, oncologists need to recognize that their decisions dictate costs. Second, doctors and patients both need to have more realistic expectations. Third, reimbursement needs to value management rather than just medication delivery. Fourth, palliative care (hospice) needs to be maximized. And fifth, cost-effectiveness must be factored into decision-making.

Cancer treatment is just one aspect of complicated decisions related to the costs and benefits of all medical care. Allocation of resources is always necessary, despite an aversion to such terms as "rationing." The fact remains, however, that there will always be a collision between unlimited demands (whether they be individual or corporate) and limited resources (either personal or national.) Our decisions regarding cancer care, as with all medical treatments, needs to be enhanced with knowledge not just of the potential benefits, but of the individual and social costs as well. As always, *primum non nocere* (first, do no harm), should remain the physicians mantra.

Smith, TJ and BE Hillner. Bending the Cost Curve in Cancer Care. N Engl J Med 2011; 364 (21): 2060-2065.

http://www.cancer.org/treatment/findingandpayingfortreatment/managinginsuranceissues/the-cost-of-cancer-treatment

http://www.nih.gov/news/health/jan2011/nci-12.htm

http://www.cancer.gov/aboutnci/servingpeople/cancer-statistics/costofcancer

CHAPTER III
INFECTIOUS AND SEXUALLY
TRANSMITTED DISEASES

A. THE ABC'S OF INFLUENZA

Influenza is an RNA virus that affects both humans and animals and exists in three strains: A, B, and C. Influenza A is further divided into sub-types based on surface proteins. These proteins are Hemagglutinins (H) and Neuraminidases (N). There are many variants of both of these proteins, including H1N1 and others such as H5N1, H3N2, and others. These proteins are subject to constant mutations, which enable the viruses to outwit their host's immunity. It also means that new vaccines against the flu must be developed every year based on the prevailing subtypes and their antigenic properties. Influenza B has no subtypes and Influenza C is a mild cold-like illness.

Seasonal flu is just that, seasonal. It starts in the fall (around September) and ends in the spring (around March). Normally, there are no flu cases from April to August in the Northern Hemisphere, but in 2009, the Novel H1N1 ("Swine Flu") originated in Mexico and rapidly spread around the world. The World Health Organization declared a pandemic on June 11, 2009 because it satisfied their pandemic criteria (i.e. a new virus, with human to human transmission, occurring in various locations around the world) and announced the end of the pandemic on August 11, 2010. Severity is not included in the pandemic definition and the Novel H1N1 did not appear to be any more severe than seasonal flu. In fact, 35,000 people die each year in the United States from complications of seasonal flu and only around 12,000 died due to Novel H1N1. After 2010, some of the flu cases continued to be H1N1, while others were H3N2 and other strains.

Each year, a new vaccine is developed for the seasonal flu. The vaccines available in 2010, 2011, 2012 and 2013 contained the H1N1 component, as well as H3N2 and Influenza B. Because of mortality associated with seasonal flu, the CDC recommendation is currently that everyone older than six months be vaccinated. Priority populations for flu vaccination still include (1) pregnant women, (2) children from 6 months to five years, (3) people 50 years of age and older, (4) people of any age with chronic medical conditions, (5) residents of nursing homes and other long-term care facilities and

(6) those who live with or care for others at high risk for influenza including health care workers, household contacts of those at high risk for flu and caregivers of children less than 6 months old. The flu shot (inactivated vaccine) is approved for anyone 6 months and older. The nasal spray flu (live attenuated influenza vaccine) is approved for healthy people 2-49 who are not pregnant.

Treatment of flu remains largely symptomatic unless the patient belongs to a high risk group. Antiviral medications must be given within 48 hours of contracting symptoms to be effective. Medications may shorten the course of the illness by only a day or two in otherwise healthy individuals. Since you can "hear flu spreading," those with sneezing, coughing, and fever, with or without body aches and nausea, should stay at home until they have not had fever for 24 hours. Cough in your sleeve, not your hand. Wash your hands often or use hand sanitizer, especially in public places.

Knowing the ABCs of Influenza might not make you feel much better when you are sick, but it might help you from becoming sick in the first place.

www.cdc.gov/flu

B. PERTUSSIS (WHOOPING COUGH): THE RETURN OF OLD ENEMY

Pertussis (or Whooping Cough) is caused by *Bordetella pertussis* and has long been a vaccine-preventable disease. Coughing or sneezing easily transmits the germ, which can have deadly consequences, especially in children less than six months of age. An initial cold-like "catarrhal" stage leads to irritation and inflammation of the respiratory tract and eventually to a "paroxysmal" stage with episodes of violent coughing. Problems inhaling result in the characteristic "whoop" as the infant or child struggles to take in air. Fifty percent of infected children less than one year of age will require hospitalization, while 1 in 20 will develop pneumonia and 1 in 100 will have convulsions. A few will die (18 in the U.S. in 2008).

Pertussis tends to occur cyclically, peaking every 3 to 5 years as the immunity wears off in a significant segment of the population. More than 25,000 cases were reported in 2005, the last peak year. And since many previously vaccinated adults may get a mild form of the disease, the numbers are probably much higher. Around 900 cases were reported in California in 2010, with 5 infant deaths.

Since almost all children are vaccinated as infants (at 2, 4, and 6 months of age and again at 15-18 months of age and 4-6 years of age), you might wonder why this disease continues to claim lives throughout the United States. One problem is with very young children who have not completed their vaccination program and still remain susceptible. The other problem is that older adolescents and adults gradually lose their immunity and can contract pertussis as a cold-like disease with a nagging cough. These individuals in turn can infect incompletely vaccinated infants.

The solution has been the development and use of Tdap (Tetanos, diphtheria and Pertussis), a vaccine destined for adolescents and adults. Pre-teens getting their checkup at 11-12 years should have a dose of Tdap. Adults 19-64 who did not get a Tdap as a pre-teen should receive a dose of Tdap instead of their next regular tetanus booster. By vaccinating adolescents and adults, increased immunity helps prevent adult caregivers and siblings from contracting the disease and transmitting it to susceptible infants.

Even though the vaccine is highly effective, it does not offer 100% immunity and some people may still be infected with pertussis, albeit in a mild version. People with a cough should always keep away from very young infants, especially those one year or younger.

Since this unwelcome germ is still among us, be sure to get your Tdap when you get your next tetanus booster. Encourage all parents to vaccinate their children and stay away from young infants if you have a cough or cold. If you have a chronic, persistent cough, make sure your doctor considers the possibility of pertussis. We may not be able to eliminate this troublesome infection, but we can try to blunt its impact in our communities, especially among that vulnerable population of children one year old or less.

www.cdc.gov/pertussis/

C. MEASLES: RETURN OF AN OLD FOE

Many people only remember measles as a childhood disease of their grandparents. While measles still routinely exists in the wild in many areas of the world, it was declared as "eliminated" in the United States in 2000. That meant there were no longer any year-round local cases.

In 2011, nonetheless, 222 cases and 17 measles outbreaks (three or more cases related in time and place) were reported in the United States. Most of these cases were imported from other countries, 52 in U.S. residents traveling overseas and 20 in foreign visitors, but the others occurred in unvaccinated Americans who were exposed to one of those two groups. Although the numbers are very small, there is still potential for more serious outbreaks given the extreme contagiousness of the disease and the existence of a small, but persistent group of unvaccinated Americans.

The problem is not that the vaccine does not work. On the contrary, one dose results in over 90% coverage when given to children between 19 and 35 months of age. Certain people, however, decline vaccinations for themselves and for their children due to religious beliefs or unfounded health concerns. Few people remember the ravages caused by measles, which results in rare but devastating cases of encephalitis, with permanent neurological damage and occasional deaths. In Europe, where vaccination is general (albeit incomplete in some countries) there were still over 30,000 cases of measles reported in 2011, with 27 cases of meningo-encephalitis and eight deaths.

Because of the persistence of un-vaccinated clusters and the rapid spread of the disease, it should always be considered in a febrile child with a generalized maculo-papular rash, often associated with cough, conjunctivitis and a runny nose. Travel abroad or association with foreign travelers should increase suspicion. Isolations precautions should be started immediately and any suspected case reported to the Office of Public Health. Disease surveillance specialists in the Infectious Disease Department will contact the CDC, which works closely with local health departments. Prompt reporting and isolation allows outbreaks to be limited in size.

All children should receive an MMR (Measles, Mumps and Rubella) vaccination at 12-15 months, with a second dose at between 4-6 years. Unvaccinated travelers, health professionals or college students should also receive two doses of MMR. Other unvaccinated adults should receive at least one MMR dose. Previously unvaccinated children over one year of age should get two MMR doses (separated by at least 28 days) prior to foreign travel.

Measles is still very much present worldwide and it remains highly contagious. Vaccines are safe and effective. Do not put yourself or your children at risk for serious complications and possible death when a couple of shots will offer almost complete protection.

CDC. Measles-United States, 2011. MMWR 2012;61(15)223-257.

www.cdc.gov/measles/index.html

D. HEPATITIS C: BOOMERS BEWARE!

Hepatitis C is a viral disease (with several genotypes), most often spread by blood exposure, which affects the liver and can cause cirrhosis and liver cancer. This insidious disease is not rare and affects over 3 million adults in the United States, most of them born between 1945 and 1965. The CDC estimates that there were 17,000 new cases in 2007 alone and over 15,000 people died from complications of hepatitis C in the same year.

So why target the baby boomers? First, testing for hepatitis C is relatively recent and only became widespread in the 1990's. Second, most people do not know they were infected and only around 25% of newly infected hepatitis C patients have jaundice, or other non-specific symptoms of fatigue, abdominal pain, joint pain, nausea and vomiting. Third, in the 1970's and 1980's, injection drug use, blood transfusions, hemodialysis (and more rarely sexual contact), all resulted in widespread hepatitis C exposures. As a result, many people were exposed and they are only now becoming identifiable and treatable.

Of exposed individuals, a lucky 20% or so clear the virus spontaneously. The remaining 80% go on to develop a chronic infection, which, in turn, will result in chronic liver disease in most of those sufferers. Over the course of 20-30 years, around 10% of infected individual will develop cirrhosis and about half of those will die of liver failure or hepatitis C-related liver cancer. In the United States today, hepatitis C remains the number one indication for liver transplants

Injectable drug use remains the leading cause of infection and around 30% of users from 18-30 years old are infected. While very high, this is much lower than the 70-90% of IV drug users in the over 30 age group. Although hepatitis C was formerly transmitted by blood transfusion, adequate screening has reduced that risk to 1 in 2 million transfused units. Infection through accidental needle sticks and perinatal transmission remains possible, although rare.

There are now readily available screening tests, which must be followed by more refined confirmatory tests (RNA polymerase chain reaction)

when the screening tests are positive. These tests become positive 1-3 months after exposure and will detect antibodies in over 97% of cases after 6 months.

Testing for all Baby Boomers has become critically important because of the large number of infected individual and the development of effective methods of treatment. Use of pegylated interferon and ribavirin (two older anti-viral treatments), associated with newer polymerase and protease inhibitors (also used in HIV infections) has greatly improved response rates. Although the individual response varies, over 50% of those infected with genotype 1 and over 80% of those infected with genotype 3 can show "sustained virologic responses" (undetectable virus in the patient's blood 6 months after completing treatment.)

Whereas hepatitis C was once undetectable and untreatable, now it is both easy to diagnosis and responsive to appropriate therapy in most individuals. Liver transplants for Hepatitis C may become a thing of the past. So all boomers (those born between 1945 and 1965) should ask about the hepatitis C blood test and medical providers should always propose it. It might save your life.

http://www.cdc.gov/hepatitis/C/index.htm

E. SEXUALLY TRANSMITTED DISEASES AND RACIAL DISPARITIES

In 2009, 2010 and 2012, Louisiana had the sad distinction of being number one (1) in the United States for rates of syphilis. Since sexually transmitted diseases (STDs) rarely travel alone, it should be of no surprise that we were also number two (2) or (3) for gonorrhea and Chlamydia and number four (4) for HIV/AIDS. Although the order may change slightly, we have remained in the top 5 for many years.

Each of these diseases creates its own problems, sometimes rather benign, such as mild genital irritation and discharge as with gonorrhea and Chlamydia. But other effects can be much more devastating and include infertility in women (gonorrhea and Chlamydia), neurological damage (syphilis), and lifelong infection with susceptibility to other diseases (HIV/AIDS).

Sexually transmitted diseases affect 15 million people each year in the United States and cost $8.4 billion in medical costs and lost wages. By age 25, one third of all sexually active young adults will have been infected by one or more STD. This national and state epidemic is, as mentioned, particularly severe in Louisiana, although we share this distinction with the neighboring states of Mississippi and Alabama, as well as other states of the Old South.

Why should this be the case? The answer lies in demographics. Although STDs represent a huge problem across the nation, it disproportionately affects the African-American community. For whatever reasons, rates for all STDs are 8 to 26 times greater among blacks than among whites or Hispanics. This translates into higher state (or parish) rates for areas with higher black populations. This situation is the undisputed reality, but it is certainly not inevitable. The statistics may be skewed by the fact that African-Americans represent a disproportionate number of patients treated by public health providers, who systematically test and report STDs. Nonetheless, striking racial disparities do exist.

One possible solution to the problem of STDs, at least in part, lies in aggressive and realistic STD education in the young adolescent population. Because some teens are sexually active at a very early age, STD education should optimally begin in junior high or even earlier. Yet there remains considerable resistance from some parents and even some schools and educators to the inclusion of specific information concerning STDs in the school setting. The subject is difficult, not only because differences in sexual development among adolescents is enormous, but also because of the delicate nature of the subject itself, complicated by unsettling racial disparities. Not discussing the issue, however, is not helpful, but only increases the burden of disease for individuals and the state.

The age of onset of sexual activity during high school nationwide varies and is highest among black males (79% of whom are sexual active before the end of high school) and lowest among Asian females (23%). The implications of this are clear, sexual education, including STDs, should occur early, especially in schools with significant African-American populations. Resistance by parents, school boards and superintendents should be expected in some circumstances, but should not be an insurmountable deterrent.

Comprehensive STD education is particularly important with HIV/AIDS because twenty-five percent of people with HIV are not aware they are infected. In addition, this disease, once considered the scourge of White gay males, is now disproportionally common among African-Americans. One of the fastest growing groups of new cases is, in fact, among black heterosexual women.

All of this may be considered unpleasant, but ignorance is not bliss and silence is not golden. Sexually transmitted diseases should be openly discussed in homes, churches and schools. Sexual education should, of course, be initiated at home. Yet parents do not always have the expertise or the inclination to address such messy matters. Not discussing STDs is, however, not acceptable. These diseases cause varying levels of misery in individuals, and the society as a whole pays the $8.4 billion dollar price tag.

Sexuality is a remarkably potent force and, like the tide, can be observed, but not successfully held back. That same tide carries both blessings and maledictions. If we learn about those undesirable elements, such as STDs, we can protect others and ourselves. Each one of us can be part of the solution or we can remain part of the problem by active collusion or by inaction.

www.cdc.gov/std/

http://new.dhh.louisiana.gov/assets/oph/HIVSTD/hiv-aids/2013/2011STDAnnualReport.pdf

F. HUMAN PAPILLOMA VIRUS (HPV): THE ENEMY WITHIN

Human Papilloma Virus (HPV) is one of many viruses that infect humans (and other primates). Viruses are bits of genetic material, housed in a capsule, that inject themselves into their human host cells. The genetic material is actually incorporated into the cell's own genetic material. In essence, the human host cell is high jacked by the virus and turned into a viral replication factory.

There are many strains of HPV, one of which is the HPV-16. Some strains are more virulent than others. The problem with HPV, as with many viruses, is that once it infects the host, it may remain there for days, months, years, or even indefinitely. So once we get high jacked, what harm does this intracellular pirate cause?

Although you may not have heard of HPV, everyone knows about *verruca vulgaris*, or common skin warts. Common warts can form on any part of the body, but are often located on the hands. They can last for months or years. They can also disappear without treatment if the body's immunity overcomes the invader. Freezing or burning them off, as long as the root is treated, can result in cure. They are, however, remarkably tenacious.

Condyloma accuminata, or genital warts, is the same problem, albeit in a different location. Genital warts can be huge and recurrent, despite multiple applications of a corrosive agent, TCA (trichloracetic acid.) Burning off the top genital wart sometimes reduces the size, but rarely eliminates the offending virus, which continues to live deep in the tissues and reforms the wart at a later date.

While genital warts are unpleasant, even disfiguring, the virus (especially HPV-16) has the propensity of inhibiting elements in the cell that promote the repair of damaged cellular DNA. Without these protective proteins, cells become dysfunctional and can undergo malignant (cancerous) transformation. Through this mechanism, HPV causes both cervical cancer in women and head and neck cancers in both men and women. Over 10,000 women die each year of HPV induced cervical cancers. The cost, both in lives and money, is staggering, all the more so since this is a vaccine-preventable illness.

Some years ago, a vaccine became available against HPV. The vaccine is given by pediatricians, obstetricians-gynecologists, and through the Office of Public Health. Since HPV is a sexually transmitted disease that can be treated but not cured, any preventive measures, such as vaccination, must be considered. Prevention is always the best medicine.

To be effective, the HPV vaccine is best administered prior to the initiation of sexual activity. Girls should be vaccinated after they reach 9 years of age and usually after 11, but may be vaccinated later if they have not already done so. Vaccination for HPV is approved for us in women up to 26 years of age, although it is usually completed prior to age 19. The vaccine is given in a series of three intra-muscular shots at 1, 2 and 6 months. Even after exposures to HPV, there are many strains, so vaccination, while it will not cure an existing infection, will help prevent other strains, notably the cancer-causing HPV-16.

Boys can be vaccinated as well. Although they are not subject to cervical cancer, they can contract and transmit HPV and are subject to HPV induced head and neck cancer. In addition, an infected person will spread the disease through sexual intercourse to his partner or partners. Available without charge from the Office of Public Health for some adolescents up to 19 years of age, the vaccine can cost up to $120 per shot (and three are required) at most private providers, depending on the person's insurance coverage.

In conclusion, HPV represents more than a nuisance and the vaccine should be given to adolescents, especially girls, prior to the initiation of sexual intercourse. Help your body fight HPV, this insidious high jacking pirate that causes cervical cancer and genital warts. HPV vaccine is the only vaccine known to prevent cancer, and it behooves both parents and grandparents to have their pre-adolescent and adolescent children protected.

http://www.cdc.gov/hpv/

G. LEPROSY IN LOUISIANA: A TENACIOUS PRESENCE

Leprosy evokes Biblical images of nose-less, limbless deformed outcasts, living in squalor. The fact is that leprosy, or Hansen's disease as it is officially called, has never really gone away, but has morphed into something often mild and very treatable right here in Louisiana.

Hansen's disease is caused by the *Mycobacterium leprae*, a slow-growing bacteria this is partial to the skin, mucous membranes, nerves, eyes and bones. If left unchecked, the germ damages the peripheral nerves, leaving the sufferer insensitive to pain. It is recurrent trauma and tissue destruction, rather than erosion by the bacteria itself, that lead to loss of extremities from a lack of sensation.

Leprosy has been documented in Louisiana since colonial days and was traditionally limited to the "Acadian Triangle," or the French-speaking parishes of South Louisiana and New Orleans. The number of cases increased to the point that the famous leprosarium at Carville, Louisiana, was established in 1880 and taken over by the U.S. government in 1921. From the 1930's to the 1960's, the number of cases progressively declined and stabilized, resulting in the closure of Carville as a leprosarium in the mid 1980's. From the 1960's, the downward trend, however, has been replaced by a slow but steady increase in the number of cases, notably outside of the traditional endemic region of South Louisiana.

The exact cause of this increase is not entirely clear, but may be associated with exposure to the nine-banded armadillo. The temperature of armadillo footpads is about the same as human skin and about 5-10% of these animals appear to be susceptible to leprosy. The germ grows on their footpads and can contaminate the soil and air surrounding an infected animal. Contact with armadillos, rather than with close family contacts as in the past, appears to be the only source suggested in over 50% of newly diagnosed cases.

Despite its fearsome reputation, Hansen's disease is very treatable. A simple antibiotic regimen (with Dapsone and Rifampin, with or without Clofazimine) will render the patient incapable of spreading the disease within a couple of weeks. The treatment course depends on response and can last months or years, but without institutionalization and with no risk to surrounding family, friends or co-workers.

Most leprosy cases in Louisiana are native-born citizens (94%), mostly white (77%) and male. Time to diagnosis has decreased dramatically, with most cases being diagnosed within a year of onset. The presentation varies from a few light-colored skin patches (tuberculoid) to multiple nodules, plaques and involvement of the nasal mucosa associated with stuffiness and nose bleeds (lepromatous). A skin biopsy, with special stains, confirms the diagnosis.

Because it is relatively rare, many physicians do not think about leprosy. It should always be considered in immigrants, residents of Louisiana or Texas, or those with foreign travel who present with localized patches of light-colored skin, especially if associated with thickened nerves and sensory loss. Hansen's disease, while sometimes not considered, is easy to treat when it is correctly diagnosed, and certainly not the dreaded Biblical disease of days gone by.

http://www.hrsa.gov/hansens

www.cdc.gov/leprosy/

http://www.dhh.louisiana.gov/assets/oph/Center-PHCH/Center-CH/infectious-epi/EpiManual/LeprosySummary.pdf

http://www.ncbi.nlm.nih.gov/pmc/articles/PMC2239329/

http://www.dhh.louisiana.gov/assets/oph/Center-PHCH/Center-CH/infectious-epi/Annuals/LaIDAnnual_Leprosy.pdf

H. RABIES: THE BITES THAT KILL

Rabies is a disease of animals caused by a virus of the genus *Lyssavirus*. Although it is present in many species of wild animals, notably skunks, raccoons, bats, and foxes, it also can affect dogs, cats, and even deer and cattle. The reservoir species, those in which the disease occurs regularly, can transmit the disease to any warm-blooded animal, including humans, through saliva from a bite.

Although the number of cases of rabies in humans in the United States is very small (4 cases in 2009 and 2 in 2010), untreated rabies is almost always fatal. Worldwide, it is estimated that 55,000 people are killed by rabies each year. Since the initiation of regular vaccination among dogs and cats in the United States, the number of cases in domestic animals has dropped dramatically and is now largely exceeded by cases in wildlife (92% in 2010).

Within wildlife populations, there are rabies virus variants typical of the host animal, but communicable to other species. Of the over 6,000 rabies cases reported in the United States in 2010, the percentages varied as follows: raccoons (36.5%), skunks (23.5%), bats (23.2%), foxes (6.9%), cats (4.9%), cattle (1.1%) and dogs (1.1%). The distribution of infected wild animals varies significantly, with raccoon being infected on the East Coast, foxes in the Southwest (and Alaska), and skunks scattered around the West, Southwest, Central and Southern U.S. Bats have a much wider, scattered distribution and rabid bats can occur in almost any state, with a special concentration in Southeast Texas.

Once bitten, the onset of symptoms from rabies varies with the site of the inoculation. Since the virus travels up the nerves to the brain, bites in the extremities are much slower to manifest themselves then bites to the face (where the distance to the brain is much shorter.) Early signs include headache and fever, followed eventually (in weeks or months) by confusion, hallucinations, hyper-salivation, hydrophobia (fear of water), and ultimately, death. Timely delivery of prophylactic medications, which includes Rabies Immune Globulin at the site of the bite and Rabies Vaccine IM at days 0, 3, 7 and 14, will stop the progression of the disease. Deaths in humans result from delays in seeking medical assistance, usually because the victim is unaware of the initial bite (as might occur from a bat.)

Despite the few cases of rabid domestic animals, dog and cat bites still occur very frequently, somewhere between 1.5 and 3.5 million a year. Almost 1% of animal bites treated in emergency rooms require hospitalization. If the dog, cat or other animal cannot be located, or has no documented history of up-to-date rabies vaccination, then rabies prophylaxis (immune globulin and vaccine) should always be recommended, despite the cost of over $1,000. An alternative is to quarantine the animal for ten days and if any signs of rabies develop, to sacrifice the animal and have its brain examined at the State Laboratory of the Office of Public Health. All wild animals should be considered rabid and prophylaxis initiated unless they can be captured, euthanized and tested.

A terrible dilemma occurs when the animal is a beloved pet that has bitten a child on the face, and prophylaxis should not be delayed. The owner must make the painful decision of inflicting medical treatment on the child or sacrificing the animal for a more rapid answer to the question of rabies infection. Up-to-date vaccinations in all pets would make such a heartbreaking choice unnecessary.

To prevent rabies from killing animals (or people), always vaccinate your pets, keep them from wild animals, report strays and enjoy wildlife from a distance. For children, "Love your own pets, leave others alone" should be the rule. If you travel, remember that rabies is still very common worldwide and you should never pet stray dogs on the roadside in some distant village. Getting correctly treated for rabies prophylaxis in such circumstances could prove difficult or impossible.

www.worldrabiesday.org

www.cdc.gov/rabies

http://www.dhh.louisiana.gov/assets/oph/Center-PHCH/Center-CH/infectious-epi/Annuals/LaIDAnnual_Rabies.pdf

I. NAEGLERIA FOWLERI: THE "BRAIN-EATING" AMOEBA

A rash of recent deaths from the so-called "brain-eating" amoeba, *Naegleria fowleri*, has galvanized the press and public opinion in Louisiana. Although these cases are exceedingly rare, with only three deaths since 2011 in Louisiana (31 cases in the U.S. from 2003-2012), their severity, sometimes resulting in the death of a child, strikes fear into the heart of every parent. What is this "brain-eating" menace to public health? Where does it come from? And how can it be treated or prevented?

Advances in water treatment over the last century (at least in the United States and other developed countries) have almost eliminated water-borne scourges of the past such as typhoid fever and cholera. Deadly epidemics of these diseases led to an awareness of the importance of clean drinking water to public health and rapid improvements in treatment techniques. We have all grown used to viewing safe water as a fact of life. Any potentially deadly organism in our drinking water disturbs our sense of security and *Naegleria fowleri* is no exception.

Naegleria fowleri, is a microscopic one-celled animal called an amoeba. These creatures change their shape continuously to move around, surrounding and ingesting the particulate matter they consume. Although this organism normally lives in warm fresh water, and is destroyed by stomach acid when ingested, a problem occurs when it finds itself in the wrong place. If one of these amoebas gets deep into the nasal cavity, it can come in contact with the cribriform plate. This is a very thin perforated bone that separates the nasal cavity from the brain. Since this plate is covered only be a thin layer of tissue on both sides, the amoeba can change shapes and literally squeeze through the perforated bone and get directly into the brain. *Naegleria fowleri* destroys normal brain tissue as it multiples in the warm, nutrient rich surroundings of the central nervous system, thus its "brain-eating" reputation. Unchecked, it can cause severe damage or death, as has occurred in several well reported cases.

Treatment requires prompt identification of the organism and use of special anti-infectious agents, some of which are experimental. If the patient does not die, they often require long-term life support in the intensive care unit to overcome the illness.

Since we all drink water and occasionally get it into our noses, and since *Naegleria fowleri* is naturally occurring and widespread in the environment, why don't more people come down with the disease? First, water treatment with chlorine (or chloramines) should result in residual chlorine levels (0.5 mg/L) that kill the organism. Water system operators monitor these levels and reports are sent to the Department of Health and Hospitals for review. There are, however, over 1,300 water systems scattered throughout the state, with variations in size, complexity, distribution and water source (surface or underground), which makes the task challenging.

Second, despite the ubiquitous presence of *Naegleria fowleri*, we usually only drink or bathe in tap water, without getting it up our nose. The intentional nasal intake of water with Neti pots or other devices for "cleansing the sinuses," can put the organism in the wrong place and should only be done with distilled water as recommended by the manufacturers. Children and adults should avoid getting water up their noses, especially in natural bodies of water, backyard pools and water parks. Maintaining adequate chlorination under such circumstances becomes difficult, if not impossible, so prevention is the best medicine. That being said, a recent emergency rule from the Department of Health and Hospitals requires more frequent testing of water systems and strict adherence to the requirement of residual chlorine levels of at least 0.5 mg/L.

Clean, safe drinking water is still the rule. Many competent professionals, from your local water system operators to state surveillance personnel, work very hard to guarantee water quality and safety. Yet it is still almost impossible to assure a totally safe and sterile environment, especially in natural bodies of water. We share the planet with a host of friendly and not-so-friendly animals and plants. Learn to recognize friend from foe among our neighbors and keep water out of your nose. That being said, your tap water is safe drink, so enjoy a big glass.

http://www.cdc.gov/parasites/naegleria/general.html

http://www.dhh.louisiana.gov/index.cfm/newsroom/detail/2870

J. LYME DISEASE: TICK-BOURNE TROUBLE

Lyme disease, first described by Dr. Willy Burgdorfer in 1892, has evoked a tremendous amount of interest in the scientific and lay press. The disease, caused by a spirochete, *Borrelia burgdorferi*, occurs in certain host animals, such as the white-tailed deer, and can be transmitted to humans through the bite of the infected deer tick (or black legged tick), *Ixodes scapularis*. As anyone who enjoys the outdoors knows, ticks are extremely common, and the deer tick is found throughout the East, South and Western Great Lakes regions in the United States.

If bitten by an infected tick, there is a 3 day to one month incubation period, followed by the appearance of a typical bull's eye-like rash up to 20 inches in diameter known as "erythema migrans" (or migrating red rash). Fever, headache, fatigue and muscular and joint pains often accompany this rash. If the disease is identified, the patient can receive a two to four week course of antibiotics (either doxycycline or amoxicillin) with complete resolution of the disease.

There are laboratory tests for Lyme disease whose interpretations are very problematic for patients outside of the limited endemic areas mentioned above. For those with a clear history of tick exposure and clear symptomatology (from the appropriate geographical regions), a screening test (ELISA or enzyme-linked immunosorbant assay) and confirmatory test (Western Blot) are both required. There are other screening tests, including the ILA (Immunofluorescent assay), C6 and PreVue *B. burgdorferi* Antibody Detection Assay. Unfortunately, the multiplicity of tests, especially when performed in those with a low probability of disease, leads to numerous false-positive diagnoses (meaning the patient does not really have Lyme disease.) About 5% of the general population will have a false positive IgM Western Blot, sometimes caused by common viruses (Cytomegalovirus, Epstein-Barr virus, Varicella-Zoster or Herpes Simplex) or rheumatoid arthritis, lupus or syphilis. In addition, the CDC or the Infectious Diseases Society of America (IDSA) does not recognize some laboratory tests as being valid for making a definitive diagnosis of Lyme disease. Over-diagnosis is, therefore, a rampant problem.

One curiosity about the proliferation of purported Lyme disease is that it does not follow the disease's true geographic distribution. While the deer tick is found all over the Eastern and Southern United States, true cases of Lyme disease are densely concentrated in the Northeast and the Western Great Lakes region. Rare cases have been reported elsewhere, often related to travel to endemic areas. The exact explanation for this limited geographical disease distribution is unclear, although it felt the tick might feed on non-deer hosts that do not transmit the disease outside of the limited Northern concentrations. Under any circumstances, it is best to avoid ticks since they carry a number of other diseases, notably Rocky Mountain spotted fever, which is found in the Mid-Atlantic and Southern states as well.

Aggravating the difficulties of making a correct diagnosis, there has been a proliferation of providers specializing in the treatment of a so-called "Chronic Lyme Disease," an entity that has no basis in medical fact. A whole group of self-described "Lyme Literate Medical Doctors" (LLMDs) has emerged and has promulgated their own "Official Guidelines" (not recognized by the CDC or IDSA) for treatment of Chronic Lyme Disease. Such physicians may recommend treatments that are unproven and unsafe, including Malaria therapy, intracellular hyperthermia therapy with DNP (2,4-dinitrophenol), hyperbaric oxygen therapy, colloidal silver, electromagnetic "rife machines," and injections with hydrogen peroxide or bismacine.

Some LLMDs, use prolonged, recurrent courses of IV antibiotics, including ceftriaxone, which can provoke gallstones and sometimes result in line-associated sepsis. Some sufferers become "antibiotic addicts," who insist on repeated courses of IV and oral antibiotics, even as the risks of such treatments exceed the purported benefits. Recurrent antibiotic use can cause a constellation of uncomfortable symptoms, including fever, chills, tachycardia and muscle aches. These "Jarish-Herxheimer Reactions," popularly called "herxing," are actually accepted and requested by certain patients who feel that suffering is necessary to achieve a cure. All such unsubstantiated treatments have caused harm to some patients, including death, and have resulted in the subsequent sanctioning of practitioners, up to and including loss of licensure, fines and jail time.

Fortunately, true Lyme disease and most other tick-borne diseases are readily treated with oral antibiotics. Lyme disease does not remain indefinitely in the body and the myth of "Chronic Lyme disease" should be put to rest. Unexplained symptoms frustrate patients, especially if they cannot get what they consider to be a reasonable explanation. Sufferers may seek an unreasonably explanation, which they sometimes defend with great passion on the Internet and elsewhere. A complicit practitioner, therefore, becomes part of the problem, not part of the solution.

http://www.cdc.gov/lyme/

http://new.dhh.louisiana.gov/assets/oph/Center-PHCH/Center-CH/infectious-epi/Annuals/LaIDAnnual_Lyme.pdf

http://www.quackwatch.org/01QuackeryRelatedTopics/lyme.html

K. CLOSTRIDIUM DIFFICILE:
A DEADLY AND DIFFICULT INFECTION

Clostridium difficile, as its name implies, is a very difficult germ. "Difficile," the Latin word for "difficult," comes from the fact that it is hard to culture in the lab, but that is the least of our worries. Although it is a naturally occurring germ (found in the stool of 3% of healthy adults), it can cause serious diarrhea and even death, especially in the elderly who are hospitalized or are residents of nursing homes or long term care facilities.

It is estimated that *Clostridium difficile* (or "C diff" as it is often called) causes over 500,000 cases of acute diarrheal disease and contributes to 28,000 deaths each year in the United States alone. New cases of *Clostridium difficile* infection (CDI) have steadily increased over the past decades and now cause around 25% of all hospital-acquired diarrheas. It adds anywhere from 3 to 20 days to a hospital stay and costs more than a billion dollars in additional health care costs each year.

What is this terrible germ? It is a spore-forming microbe that lives in places without oxygen, such as the human gut. It is excreted in fecal matter, which can contaminate the environment, especially in health care settings. In normal individuals, it usual causes no disease since our guts are full of "good bacteria," which neutralize the growth of *Clostridium*. But in those who have taken antibiotics, the good germs are greatly reduced and *Clostridium* can proliferate. It produces toxins that inflame the gut (causing colitis) and provoking massive diarrhea, abdominal pain, fever and occasionally perforation of the gut and death.

Toxins from the germ can be identified in the stool and lead to the diagnosis. Several methods exist, but the enzyme immunoassay is one of the most common and quickest tests. Like most tests, it is not 100% accurate and can give both false positive and false negative results. Multiple tests are sometimes necessary to confirm the diagnosis.

Treatment can be as simple as stopping the offending antibiotic and many cases resolve in 2-3 days. If not, there are special oral antibiotics (either metronidazole or vancomycin) that can be used. Some patients require multiple treatments to completely clear the germ from their gut. Severe cases may require hospitalization and even surgical removal of the bowel.

One of two disturbing recent developments has been the emergence of a "hyper virulent" strain of *C. difficile* (BI/NAP 1/027). This strain causes double the mortality of the usual strain and has spread around the world. The other disturbing trend has been the emergence of Community-acquired *C. difficile* in the general healthy population, who may not have been exposed to antibiotics and who are not considered high risk populations (children, young adults and woman after childbirth).

Once established in an environment, the spores of *C. difficile* are resistant to drying and even to alcohol. Contamination of a hospital or nursing home room becomes very hard to eradicate. New residents of contaminated room may be infected or re-infected by exposure to the residual spores.

So how do we protect ourselves from this threat? There are a few simple things we can do to significantly reduce the risk: (1) Do not use antibiotics unless they are necessary. (2) Wash your hands, especially in the hospital or nursing home and be sure all health care providers do the same. (3) If you have a severe diarrhea lasting more than three days, seek medical advice. (4) If you are in a place where someone is or has been ill with *C. difficile*, make sure the entire area has been cleaned with diluted bleach. (Remember, neither soap nor alcohol kills the spores, which survive in the environment for days or weeks.)

As you can see, *Clostridium* is indeed a "difficult" problem, which requires the full collaboration of both the general public and healthcare providers to resolve. For more information about *C. difficile*, please consult www.cdc.gov or www.mayoclinic.com.

www.cdc.gov/HAI/organisms/cdiff/Cdiff_infect.html

L. METHICILLIN RESISTANT STAPH AUREUS
(MRSA or "MERSA")

Almost everyone has heard of Methicillin Resistant Staph Aureus (MRSA or "MERSA") these days. As a source of boils in high school or college athletes or the cause of devastating complications in hospitalized patients, MRSA seems to be everywhere.

In fact, *Staphylococcus aureus* is a germ that lives on the skin of over 30% of healthy people. It, like many other bacteria, was once universally sensitive to penicillin. Within a few years of the development of penicillin in 1940, some resistant strains had already been identified. Other antibiotics were subsequently invented, including methicillin in 1960, but by 1963, resistance to methicillin had also developed. Resistance continued to extend to other antibiotics until multi-resistant *Staphylococcus* became a worldwide epidemic. By 2010, over 60% of all hospital strains of *Staphylococcus* were MRSA, and some had become resistant to Vancomycin, one of the mainstays of treatment.

MRSA is not only widespread in hospitals but has gradually spilled out into the general community. Staphylococcal strains are now divided into HA-MRSA (Hospital Associated) and CA-MRSA (Community Associated.) The latter was further divided into strains associated with healthcare institutions (nursing homes, for example) and those that appear spontaneously in the community. Wherever MRSA comes from and however it manifests itself, it still represents a terrific medical challenge.

In Louisiana, about 1.5 million people (30% of the populations) are colonized with *Staphylococcus*, while only about 1% (or 45,000) carries MRSA. This still results in countless outpatient medical visits for those unlucky enough to develop boils, cellulitis, folliculitis, or more invasive infections including pneumonia or sepsis. Although such major complications are rare in the community, over 125,000 people will develop Hospital Associated MRSA each year in the U.S. and over 5,000 will die. MRSA complications in the hospital add over 9 days to the average stay, $20,000 to the individual bill and over 4 billion dollars in aggregate costs. It is estimated that all costs associated with MRSA, both in and out of the hospital, exceed 34 billion dollars/year.

So how can we prevent ourselves from this modern day scourge? Since *Staphylococcus aureus* is everywhere, we can start by reducing the 5 C's: CONTACT, CROWDING, sharing CONTAMINATED items, covering COMPROMISED skin (open lesions) and promoting CLEANLINESS. It is imperative that all healthcare workers and visitors wash their hands prior to entering and when leaving a patient's room. Hospitals are very much attuned to the human and economic costs of MRSA (and other hospital-acquired infections). Each hospital has an Infection Control Officer who tracks such infections, reporting certain types of infections not only to their own medical institution, but also to the National Healthcare Safety Network (NHSN). There are also active programs of bacterial surveillance and isolation associated with all such cases in the hospital setting. And strict adherence to such programs along with corrective actions dramatically reduces hospital acquired MRSA cases.

On an individual level, the importance of hand washing cannot be overstated. Use of soap and water (or alcohol based hand sanitizers) reduces bacterial contamination by over 90%. Never share personal hygiene items and cover open wounds. *Staphylococcus* is here to stay and has outwitted our best attempts to develop antibiotics. This being said, judicious use of antibiotics reduces the development of resistant strains of all bacteria. If you do not really need antibiotics, don't insist on their use. Doctors, patients, hospitals, pharmaceutical companies and the general public all share the responsibility for reducing the terrible cost of this omnipresent enemy.

www.cdc.gov/mrsa/

M. HOSPITAL ACQUIRED INFECTIONS: THE UNWANTED COMPLICATION

Everyone going into the hospital hopes to get better. Surrounded by competent professionals and sophisticated technology, it seems a foregone conclusion that improvement must follow. Unfortunately, the hospital is a concentration of very sick people in a relatively small place. With sick people come germs and with germs come diseases.

Hospital acquired infections (HAIs) include catheter associated urinary tract infections, surgical site infections, ventilator associated infections, central line associated infections, Methicillin-resistant *Staphylococcus aureus* and *Clostridium difficile*. Together, they cause over 2,000 deaths a year in Louisiana, which cost around $360 million. Nationwide, the CDC states that between five and 10 percent of patients who go into the hospital will get at least one hospital acquired infection. That amounts to over 1.7 million infections and over 90,000 deaths every year, costing around $33 billion.

With such grim statistics, it would seem better to stay out of the hospital all together. Yet hospitals deliver life-saving treatments every day to the sickest of the sick and hospital administrators are well aware of the potential risks of hospital acquired infections.

Since this problem has developed along with increased resistance to antibiotics, it represents a real challenge to the medical community. Most hospitals track their hospital acquired infection rates and report them to the National Healthcare Safety Network (NHSN), a service of the Centers for Disease Control (CDC). Recommendations exist through the CDC and other organizations to implement techniques and protocols aimed at reducing the risk of introducing and spreading unwanted germs.

Improved protocols for the placement of central lines (large IV lines that go into centrally located veins) in intensive care units have resulted in reduced infections rates for *Staphylococcus* (down 73%), *Enterococcus* (down 55%), Candida (down 46%) and other gram-negative germs (down 37%). In total, these types of infections have been reduced by 58% over the last few years, a tremendous saving in human suffering and cost.

Similar campaigns have been directed toward reducing catheter associated and surgical site infections. Among other things, improved techniques involve stricter adherence to the most elementary of sanitary gestures, hand washing. Within the walls of the hospital, just as in the school gymnasium or at home, our own hands transmit most harmful germs. Adequate hand washing (over 20 seconds) with soap and water, or the use of alcohol-based gels when soap and water are not available, reduce the presence of germs by 90%. In the hospital, whether it is the doctor, the nurse, the clerical staff or the janitor, every employee and volunteer must adhere to the same strict hand washing rules.

As a patient or a visitor, your responsibility is to not bring additional germs into the hospital. And, once there, make sure that you and everyone around you takes the time and effort to wash their hands. It's a small gesture that may have enormous consequences for you or one of your loved ones.

www.cdc.gov/hai/

CHAPTER IV
EAT, DRINK AND BE SICK

A. THE WHITE MENACE: SALT AND SUGAR

The Western Diet has gradually increased the proportion of processed foods over the last several decades. Processed foods include all products that are no longer in their natural state. This includes lunchmeats, pre-prepared meals, pickles, sauces, chips, pastries, soups and many more items. While processing decreases some nutritional elements, such as vitamins, it does have the advantage of prolonging shelf life. It also offers the distinct advantage of timesaving for harried consumers in our hectic world.

Yet as the saying goes, there is no such thing as a free lunch. There is a sinister tradeoff for perceived advantages of convenience and prolonged shelf life. In response to public demand and taste, the caloric content of processed foods has increased along with their salt content. The amount of salt consumed by 90% of Americans now largely exceeds our daily requirement. Oddly enough, bread, the staff of life, is one of the leading culprits, followed by processed meats, pizza, poultry, packaged soups, cheese, prepared pasta and assorted snacks (including our notorious potato chips.) Restaurant foods, including fast foods, are particularly salt-laden.

You might say that this makes no difference. But the average American consumes over 3,000 milligrams of sodium a day, three times what they require, and the body simply cannot handle the excess. African Americans, anyone older than fifty, those already with high blood pressure or diabetes, or those with kidney disease are particularly vulnerable. Salt attracts fluid and the result is excessive strain on the blood vessels, which, over time, harden and develop chronic arteriosclerosis and subsequent hypertension. Untreated high blood pressure predisposes to increased heart disease, stroke and renal failure, costing over 20 billion dollars in medical costs a year.

Salt, however, is not the only white menace. Sugar represents the other significant health threat. Many staple foods, including rice, potatoes, wheat and corn, contain starch, a polysaccharide, which is broken down into sugar in the body. The caloric content of rice, bread and potatoes, while less per gram than fats, make up a large portion of the usual diet. Sugars, whether they come directly as processed sugar or indirectly from the breakdown of starches, require insulin to be transported into the cells. Although we usually can produce adequate amounts of insulin (except in those people with Type I diabetes), our capacity to produce insulin is limited. When our needs for insulin exceed our body's capacity to produce it, blood sugar levels rise and the result is Type II diabetes. The number of diabetic Americans has steadily increased along with obesity, which now affects 30% of the adult population.

Doctors have jokingly counseled their patients that "if it tastes good, spit it out." To some extent, that holds true. What can also be said it that "if it's white, don't eat it." That includes salt and sugar (and starches). Although they do not attack the body in the same way, both salt and sugar (the result of starch metabolism) put stresses and strains on the body that results in the devastating health problems discussed above. So, before you buy those processed foods, check the labels. If the sodium content exceeds 200 mg, think twice. In addition, put down the saltshaker, avoid concentrated sweets and maintain a healthy weight. Don't eat yourself into an early grave as so many have already done.

www.cdc.gov/salt/

www.cdc.gov/Features/Sodium/index.html

http://www.nature.com/ejcn/journal/v61/n1s/full/1602939a.html

B. NOROVIRUS, OR
HOW TO WRECK A CRUISE

Imagine that your dream trip to the Caribbean turns into a nightmare of incoercible diarrhea, nausea, vomiting and abdominal pain. Yes, this does happen and more often than you might think.

The culprit of such a scenario usually turns out to be a norovirus. It is a very hardy and highly contagious single-stranded RNA virus that can infect humans after a very small exposure. It only takes 10-100 viral particles to cause an infection, which manifests itself after 24 to 48 hours with an acute onset of watery diarrhea. There is often associated vomiting, especially in children, as well as abdominal pain and low grade fever.

Although patients may think they might die, it is rarely fatal except in very young children and the debilitated elderly, and in those cases it is due to severe dehydration. Once infected, about 30% of individuals do not have symptoms, but they can still spread the virus by fecal contamination. In the other 70%, symptoms usually last one to five days, although the patient may remain contagious up to a week after onset of diarrhea.

Norovirus is so common that it accounts for over 50% of all cases of food borne gastroenteritis and around 96% of non-bacterial cases. The virus can be identified in the stool using RT-PCR (Real-time Polymerase Chain Reaction), as the Louisiana State Epidemiologist, Dr. Raoult Ratard puts it, "the proof is in the poop." The organism is usually not present in sufficient quantities to identify it in contaminated food.

Outbreaks most commonly occur in restaurants and with catered meals (36%), nursing homes (23%), schools (13%) and vacation settings, including cruises (10%). Cruise ships provide a perfect site for Norovirus outbreaks, with a captive population in close living quarters and a very contagious organism. Despite aggressive cleaning, up to 12 successive outbreaks have been reported in the same ship.

Norovirus is remarkably resistant. It withstands temperatures from freezing to 140 degrees Fahrenheit (60 degrees Celsius). Hypochlorite in high concentrations (1000 parts per million) can be used for cleaning, as can a 10% solution of household bleach. Double strength phenolics may be effective, but cannot be used in nurseries or food preparation areas. Lysol is not effective. Aggressive hand washing with soap and water or ethanol-based hand rubs reduces infective organisms on the hands by over 90% and is always recommended.

Outbreaks in institutions, including hospitals and nursing homes, require the use of patient isolation (or at least sequestration with other infected individuals), as well as strict control of movement of both visitors and staff. Gowns and gloves need to be used and infected staff must be placed on off-duty status until at least 48 hours after resolution of symptoms.

So how do you make sure your next cruise will not be the cruise from hell? There are no absolute guarantees, but you can verify with the cruise operator that your vessel has not been contaminated in the recent past. If an outbreak should occur, wash your hands as often as practical. Most ships will have alcohol-based hand sanitizers readily available. If you should fall ill, the ship's doctor will relegate you to your cabin where you will need to drink abundant fluids for the few days of acute illness. Remember, you can remain infective for up to a week after illness, so take precautions to avoid any fecal contamination when you are back home.

Most cruises are safe and enjoyable, as long as norovirus has not come along for the ride. So *Bon Voyage*!

www.cdc.gov/norovirus/index.html

C. A FEW BAD EGGS:
SALMONELLA POISONING

Salmonella enteritidis is one of many species of *Salmonella* that occur in nature. *Salmonella* is the most common form of bacterial food poisoning and results in around over 8,000 reported cases each year in the U.S. In 2010, there were also 2,290 hospitalizations and 29 deaths, most occurring in susceptible individuals. An outbreak of the disease associated with eggs from Iowa in 2010 was extensively reported in the news media. That outbreak resulted in around 2,000 cases in ten states and prompted product recalls of 500 million eggs.

After an incubation period of a day or two, infection with *Salmonella* results in diarrhea, abdominal pain, fever and headaches. Symptoms last up to a week, after which the person may remain contagious for a week or more. Very rarely does long-term colonization occur with *Salmonella enteritidis*. In young children and debilitated adults, antibiotics may be indicated, but most people do not require them. In fact, overuse of antibiotics contributes to resistant forms of the organism.

Poultry is a common source of *Salmonella* infection. Chickens (and turkeys) are natural hosts for the disease, which can infect up to 50% of a flock. The problem has been so persistent, especially in broilers, that the Food Safety Inspection Service instituted standards in 1996, limiting the *Salmonella* contamination rate to 20% or less of chicken carcasses. Rules and regulations at that time also included preventive measures in all aspects of poultry processing in order to reduce cross contamination and bacterial growth. The goal, however, was never to eliminate entirely the presence of *Salmonella* in commercial flocks because it occurs naturally in poultry.

The problem does not limit itself to broilers, but includes eggs as well. Eggs do not leave a sterile environment (the cloaca of the chicken where both eggs and fecal matter exit). During processing, eggs are washed in mild detergents and sanitized in 120-degree water, greatly reducing surface contamination. If the outside is clean, the problem of in-shell contamination still remains. Infected hens harbor *Salmonella* in their ovaries and excrete it into the eggs themselves. It is estimated that 1:10,000 eggs may be infected in a normal flock, resulting in 1:50 consumers begin exposed each year. That number rises significantly if a larger number of laying hens are infected.

Recognizing this problem, the Food and Drug Administration began working on rules in 2004 and implementing them in July of 2010 for the largest commercial producers (50,000 eggs or more each year). Those new rules include (1) bacteriological sampling from hen house floors and manure pits for *Salmonella*, (2) limiting access to chicken houses (3) rodent control (since rodent contaminated chicken food is a prime source of *Salmonella*) (4) cleaning and disinfecting of contaminated chicken houses and (5) strict temperature control of cleaned and stored eggs.

If a producer is found to have significant *Salmonella* contamination, they must submit 4,000 eggs (1,000 per week at two week intervals) for bacteriological control or they must divert all eggs for pasteurization for the life of the flock. You might wonder why all the hens could not be treated with antibiotics? This would, of course, not solve the long-term problem of infection and would risk, as in humans, the development of antibiotic resistant *Salmonella* species.

Much of the danger to the consumer from either eggs or chicken meat can be reduced or eliminated by compete cooking of these products. Incompletely cooked eggs (or chicken meat) can and do harbor *Salmonella* or other pathogens. If you ever have any eggs from a re-call list, either destroy them or return them to the point of sale. If you believe you have become ill from eating contaminated eggs or poultry, notify your physician and the local Office of Public Health.

It is impossible to totally sanitize the food supply, especially when the organisms occur naturally. Government regulations can and do lessen the risks to consumers, but cannot eliminate them entirely. It is up to all of us the use proper preparation, handling and storage technique to avoid becoming another unintentional victim of a bad egg.

http://www.cdc.gov/salmonella/

D. RAW OYSTERS: CAVEAT EMPTOR

Although an acquired taste, slurping down raw oysters can be a savory sensory and gastronomic delight. Oysters, whether they end up being consumed raw or cooked, represent a huge Louisiana industry. Producing over 13,000,000 pounds, with one million pounds a day being consumed across the United States, the economic impact is estimated at $30,000,000 a year.

Raw oysters are a particular delicacy, eaten with a splash of lemon, lime or hot sauce and accompanied by a gulp of your preferred alcoholic beverage. What could be more wholesome? Yet raw oysters have their darker side as well. Even though the Louisiana Department of Health and Hospital and the Louisiana Department of Wildlife and Fisheries strictly monitor the oyster beds, oysters are filter feeders and may carry some unexpected and unwelcome guests. Raw oysters can transmit at least five diseases: *Vibrio vulnificus*, *Vibrio parahaemolyticus*, Hepatitis A (Hep A or HAV), Norovirus and *Vibrio cholerae* (non-01).

Vibrio vulnificus is an organism that naturally occurs in salt or brackish waters. It is not a pollutant, but a free-living animal, that is picked up by the oyster. It is most prevalent in warmer waters, and peaks in the summer months in South Louisiana. If you contract *Vibrio vulnificus*, you can have chills, fever, nausea, blistering skin lesions or even death. The good news is that most people will not get sick, even if they are exposed. The bad news is that a significant number of people are particularly susceptible and will die. Although still rare, the CDC reports around 50 cases a year in the Gulf States alone, of which 16 are fatal. This includes specifically those with underlying livers diseases (chronic hepatitis or hemochromatosis), cancer (notably lymphomas and leukemia) or any disease (or treatment) that lowers the immune response (HIV/AIDS, cancer treatments, some rheumatologic treatments, or even chronic steroid use.)

Vibrio parahaemolyticus is a close relative to *Vibrio vulnificus* and occurs in the same salt-water environments. It is also filtered from the water by raw oysters, which can transmit it to humans with some of the same symptoms of fever, nausea, and blistering skin lesions. It is, however, less deadly and although over 4,000 cases a year may occur, only around 25 are reported, and only 1-2 are fatal.

Hepatitis A, unlike *Vibrio vulnificus* and *paraheamolyticus*, is related to contamination either of the oyster producing water or by an infected individual involved in the harvesting or processing of the oysters. Hepatitis A (HAV) is relatively common, although cases have decreased dramatically since 1995 when Hep A vaccination was introduced. If contracted, Hep A is associated with chills, fever and a debilitating jaundice that is not usually fatal. The other good news is that Hepatitis A (unlike its close relatives, Hepatitis B and C) does not cause chronic hepatitis, a complex and life-threatening condition.

Norovirus, another fecal contaminant, occasional occurs and results in episodic outbreaks discussed elsewhere in more detail. Symptoms include nausea, abdominal cramping and profuse diarrhea. It is short, self-limiting disease and rarely results in death. Even very small amounts of the virus can cause infection and its presence in Gulf waters resulted in the closure of some Louisiana beds in March 2010. Imported oysters have been found to be contaminated as well, notably those from Europe (Great Britain) and the Far East (Korea).

Last, but not least, is *Vibrio cholerae*, whose name evokes fearful images of massive outbreaks and multiple deaths, most recently in Haiti. But the *Vibrio cholerae* occasionally found in contaminated oysters is the non-01, non-toxigenic variety, which causes profuse diarrhea, but usually not death. The CDC reported only 17 cases from 2000-2010, although an oyster related outbreak occurred as recently as May 2011 in Florida.

So what are the solutions to the problems associated with this succulent delicacy? (1) Not eating raw oysters is the first and most obvious solution. Cooking at appropriate temperatures kills all of these organisms. (2) Raw oysters may be pasteurized by various temperature and pressure techniques. This, however, changes the taste according to some aficionados and requires expensive equipment that small producers cannot afford. (3) The FDA has proposed Banning raw oyster sale and consumption during summer months. This solution evoked an outpouring of protest from Louisiana producers, whose waters are already strictly regulated by the Departments of Health and Hospitals and the Wildlife and Fisheries.

In the end, the consumer must make the decision. There are mandatory warnings, specifically addressed to those with chronic liver and other immune altering disorders, posted in all sites where raw oyster are consumed. Unfortunately, consumers with such conditions may intentionally or unintentionally ignore them, putting their lives at risk.

Myths abound about using lemon juice, hot sauce and accompanying alcoholic beverages to kill deadly organisms, specifically *Vibrio vulnificus*, in raw oysters. They are just that, myths. As with so many potentially dangerous activities, eating raw oysters may be hazardous to your health. Weigh the risks and gastronomic benefits and, as the Latin saying goes, caveat emptor (buyer beware).

www.wlf.louisiana.gov/fishing/oyster-program

www.cdc.gov/vibrio/vibriov.html

http://dhh.louisiana.gov/assets/oph/Center-PHCH/Center-CH/infectious-epi/EpiManual/VibrioVulnificusPublicInfo.pdf

E. ARSENIC AND OLD APPLE JUICE: ALIMENTARY HYPE AND HAZARDS

A popular television show featured a well-known celebrity physician who revealed elevated levels of arsenic in apple juice. Views of the audience showed the shock and horror in the faces of young woman, many of whom had undoubtedly given apple juice to their children as a healthy alternative to carbonated drinks. While it is always a good idea to explore potential hazards around us, it is quite another thing to create hazards where they do not exist.

Arsenic is a semi-metal element that occurs naturally in the environment. It exists in an organic form (harmless) and an inorganic form (potentially harmful). Industrially, arsenic is mostly used as a wood preservative, but is also found in paints, dyes, some soaps, semiconductors, and is used in mining and smelting as well as agriculture. Long term ingestion of arsenic can accumulate in the body, eventually resulting in skin changes, gastrointestinal symptoms, nerve problems and increased risk for a number of different cancers.

Arsenic levels (inorganic) have long been monitored in drinking water, where it occurs as a natural or extrinsic contaminant. Since 1974, the Environmental Protection Agency must determine levels of contaminants in accordance with the Safe Drinking Water Act. The Maximum Contaminant Level (or MCL) for arsenic is 0.010 mg/L or 10 ppb (parts per billion). Contamination of drinking water occurs through erosion, agricultural runoff, and waste from glass and electronic industries. Local health departments in collaboration with the affected water systems address elevated levels, when they occur.

Apple juice can, in fact, can contain some level of arsenic. The Food and Drug Administration regularly tests domestic and imported apple juice for arsenic and other contaminants. Because of the extremely low levels of inorganic arsenic in juice, there is no established Maximum Contaminants Level as exists for drinking water. Even organic apples, grown in soils with natural levels of arsenic, will contain some level of arsenic.

In their tests, the FDA distinguishes between the organic (harmless) and inorganic (potentially harmful) forms of arsenic. Any elevated results are considered on a case-by-case basis, and appropriate steps taken when abnormal results occur. Since most juice is reconstituted from concentrates from multiple sources (domestic as well as international), tracing a problem to a particular source is a challenge. Despite difficulties, however, regular testing does occur, and elevated levels are pursued with the suppliers.

The conclusion of multiple tests by the FDA on past and current samples of apple juice has been that there is no public health threat from arsenic in this product. You are a greater risk from the water out of your faucets in certain communities than from the apple juice from your supermarket shelves. Nonetheless, the FDA issued new standards concerning arsenic and apple juice that appeared in July 2013.

Water contamination is always carefully monitored and aggressively pursued by the Office of Public Health, while the FDA continues to monitor the safety of our food. That being said, outbreaks of contaminated foods (such as cases of listeria on cantaloupes or *Cyclospora* on cilantro) do occur and they are investigated with vigor, often resulting in well-publicized product recalls.

We have many things to fear in this world, but apple juice does not appear to be one of them. Fear sells newspapers, airtime and advertising. Fear does not create a climate of careful reflection necessary to solve many of the world's pressing health problems. Calm down, take a deep breath, and have a small glass of apple juice. Remember that the danger from juices, if there is any at all, is from their high sugar content. Sugar equals calories and calories can result in obesity. That, however, is a different story with a different solution.

http://www.fda.gov/Food/ResourcesForYou/Consumers/ucm271595.htm

F. CYCLOSPORIASIS:
AN UNCOMMEN FOOD-BORNE ILLNESS

Food-borne illnesses themselves are very common, with over 48 million Americans affected annually. The causative agents vary, with the top six being *Salmonella*, *Campylobacter*, *E. coli*, *Vibrio parahaemolyticus*, *Yersinia* and *Listeria* (in decreasing order). There are, however, much more uncommon organisms, including outbreaks associated with the protozoan parasite, *Cyclospora cayetanensis*, which sickened over 600 people in the U.S. from June to October 2013. Cases occurred in 22 states, including 3 in Louisiana. The creature, a one-celled organism, is secreted in the stool of infected individuals and must sporulate (a type of activation) prior to becoming infectious. That means that the oocysts (egg-like structures) must remain out of the infected host for some time, making any direct person-to-person contamination highly unlikely.

Once the oocysts sporulate (become infectious), they are taken in by eating contaminated fruits or vegetables, notably raspberries, lettuce and cilantro. When these are eaten, there is an incubation period of one to two weeks (although sometimes shorter) in which the organisms reproduce in the small intestine. At that point, the person begins to show a combination of watery (not bloody) diarrhea, nausea, abdominal cramping and fatigue. Untreated, the disease may last several weeks and result in recurrent abdominal symptoms and weight loss until it finally goes away. Treatment with trimethoprim-sulfamethozazole (Bactrim) for a week will shorten the course of the illness.

Since the symptoms are so non-specific, the diagnosis can be missed unless *Cyclospora* testing is requested. Identification of the oocysts in the stool (by direct microscopic visualization) or the presence of a positive PCR (polymerase chain reaction) DNA test results is the definitive diagnosis. As the Louisiana State Epidemiologist, Dr. Raoult Ratard, so aptly puts it, "the proof is in the poop." Once identified, *Cyclospora* is a reportable disease and the Office of Public Health should be alerted within five working days of the diagnosis.

Although rare in the United States, *Cyclospora* is common in tropical areas of both Asia and Latin America, with most cases occurring in the spring and summer. Most U.S. cases have been in returning travelers and fecal contamination of food and water remains the source of infections whether in the U.S. or abroad. It is always critical to wash fruits and vegetables thoroughly to prevent contamination. Hand washing also remains important since dirty hands transmit many food-borne organisms, including *Cyclospora*.

www.cdc.gov/parasites/cyclosporiasis

G. FOOD POISONING:
THE UNWELCOME GUEST TO THE PARTY

Nothing will spoil a family gathering, a church picnic, or a long-awaited cruise more than food poisoning. Food borne illnesses are frequent, affecting 76 million North Americans each year. They are also a significant cause of morbidity and result in over 325,000 hospitalizations and 5,000 deaths annually. The older and sicker (or younger) the patient, the more likely they are to have a tragic outcome.

Food borne illnesses are caused by a number of agents including viruses, bacteria, vibrios and other organisms. Sometimes food poisoning is an "intoxication," where the food contains toxins already produced by the proliferation of the bacteria in the food (such as is the case with *Staphylococcus aureus*). At other times, it is poisoning by growth of the organism within the infected individual (such as Salmonella). In any case, the symptoms usually include fever, nausea, vomiting, abdominal pain and diarrhea, sometimes explosive and occasionally bloody.

Since there are so many causes of food poisoning, we will concentrate on the top ten. Viruses, especially noroviruses, top the list, causing about 50% of all cases. Noroviruses are the culprits in the famous cruise ship outbreaks of diarrheal illness, and are also responsible for the periodic closures of some Louisiana oyster beds. It requires very few viruses to cause an infection and the transmission potential is staggering, often affected a cruise ship in a matter of days.

Next in line is *Salmonella enteritidis,* causing around 60,000 cases of food poisoning a year. *Salmonella,* like *Escherichia coli, Shigella, Listeria* and *Campylobacter* (all in the top ten causes), invades the intestinal wall and causes fever, abdominal pain and diarrhea. An incubation period lasting anywhere between six hours to two days or more precedes symptoms. Symptoms may last up to a week. Poultry products are particular culprits since up to 90% of chicken carcasses are contaminated with *Campylobacter* and around 20% with *Salmonella* and *Listeria.*

Other food borne agents include *Clostridium perfringens*, *Staphylococcus aureus* and *Bacillus cereus*. All three of these (also in the top ten causes of food poisoning) produce toxins, the latter two prior to being ingested. In other words, with Staph and Bacillus, the poison is already in the food before you take a bite. Victims get sick in only a few hours after eating the food, often prepared and stored under improper conditions. Who has not heard about a church picnic or wedding that ended in digestive calamity?

Rounding out the top ten is *Vibrio parahaemolyticus* and its close cousin, *Vibrio vulnificus,* both saltwater organisms. *Vibrio parahaemolyticus* is often associated with partially cooked shrimp, and can cause an unpleasant episode of diarrhea. *Vibrio vulnificus* is found in raw oysters, and while most people can eat oysters with impunity those with severe liver disease run a life threatening risk.

So how do you protect yourself against this onslaught of food borne pathogens? Some common sense measures go a long way: (1) Do not leave food in a hot car. (2) Keep your kitchen clean, especially cutting boards (avoid wood if possible), sponges and knives. (3) Make sure your refrigerator is 40 degrees and your freezer is zero. (4) Cook red meat to 160 and poultry to 180 degrees. (5) Never leave perishable foods out of the refrigerator for more than TWO HOURS. (6) Keep cold party foods on ice (7) Heat leftovers to 165 degrees. (8) Put hot foods into small units for rapid cooling. (9) If food looks or smells strange, throw it out. (10) Wash your hands before, during and after food preparation. (Please note: All degrees are in Fahrenheit.)

Remember, a few simple precautions can keep some very unwelcome guests from spoiling your next picnic or party. *Bon appétit*!

www.cdc.gov/foodsafety/

H. KITCHEN ENTREPRENEURS AND FOOD SAFETY

There are periodically well-publicized events dealing with food safety. Part of the mission of the Office of Public Health (OPH) in Louisiana, as elsewhere in the United States, is to insure that the public is protected, as much as possible, from the ravages caused by dirty water, unsafe food, and infectious diseases.

The food and water safety issues fall under the domain of the OPH environmental services, which includes engineering services and sanitarians. Engineers review plans for larger water systems and other facilities. They also oversee water quality issues by testing water and working closely with local water districts. Our sanitarians issue permits for smaller sewage systems, as well as perform inspections for restaurants, hotels, nursing homes, day care centers, prison, and many other facilities.

There are Food and Drug Sanitarians who inspects food processing and storage facilities throughout the region (and in adjacent regions). Their work compliments that of the other sanitarians who oversee the final products and how they are prepared and presented.

From time to time, there are articles in the local papers featuring new products, the results of innovative entrepreneurs who want to sell their food to the public. One example is the sale of raccoon meat, the consumption of which is a local delicacy among certain groups. Although it is legal to kill, process and eat raccoons as a private citizen, the commercial sale of the meat is illegal. It would be legal if there were a licensed processor for raccoon meat in Louisiana (or elsewhere), but there is not. All processing plants must be inspected to insure that carcasses (whether they be fish, fowl or other meat) are properly handled. Contamination with *Salmonella*, *E. coli*, *Listeria* and other organisms can have deadly consequences. Contamination occurs periodically, even under the best of circumstances in commercially inspected facilities.

Other articles have featured various sauces, spices and relishes, all interesting and tasty regional Louisiana products. Rules for the production and sale of homemade products clearly delineate what can and cannot be done. Honey, jams and jellies, and more recently baked goods, are considered "hobby" products if the total sales are less than $5000/year. Even then, the product must be correctly labeled with (1) product name, (2) list of ingredients from the largest to the smallest component, (3) manufacturer's address and (4) respective weights (in standard metric equivalents). When sales exceed $5000/year, the product must be made in a licensed production facility.

Relishes, pickles, and other acidified products, pose special problems. To avoid the dangers of botulism and other food contamination, the canning must adhere to strict standards. First, a "Process Authority" must test the food and determine whether it is low acid food (naturally due to the food itself or artificially acidified). If it is "acidified" (for example, with the addition of vinegar), the producer must have attended a Better Processing Class (offered at LSU or elsewhere). The product must then be made in an approved processing plant, which adheres to the various FDA regulations concerning such products. Most home kitchen cooks have neither the time, money or interest in pursuing such commercialization.

None of this is intended to discourage initiative or entrepreneurship, but to insure that the food we eat, like the water we drink, does not pose a health risk to the public. Please feel free to contact the sanitarian services at the Office of Public Health for specific questions about the sale of food products. Your health and safety are our business.

www.cdc.gov/foodsafety/

CHAPTER V
MEDICATIONS, DRUGS,
TESTS AND MACHINES

A. PHARMACEUTICAL MARKETING AND MADNESS

Legitimate medications (not illegal drugs) represent a 320 billion dollar industry in the United States (2011). It represents one segment of the 2.7 trillion dollars spent each year on healthcare in the United States, and over $800 dollars/per person per year (almost twice the European average.

Advances in pharmacology have resulted in some astonishing improvements in the control of hypertension, hypercholesterolemia, infectious diseases, cancer treatment and other health problems. Decreases in heart disease deaths in the United States and elsewhere are largely a result of improved control of blood pressure, cholesterol and diabetes.

Historically, marketing of prescription medications occurred principally through direct contact between pharmaceutical representatives and physicians. Unlike many industries, the products (prescription drugs) require the active participation of the doctor, who holds what is referred to as the "power of the pen." This power has been absolute and is the reason for the tremendous allocation of personnel and resources by the pharmaceutical industry to influence physician's choice of medication.

This situation began to change in the late seventies with the advent of managed care and HMOs (Health Maintenance Organizations). More and more physicians and patients were confronted with the reality of fixed formularies. A formulary is an approved list of medications from which the physician can choose. The use of generic medications, those no longer under patent and usually less expensive, is encouraged by reduced or no co-pays. Other more expensive brand name medications may be on the formulary, but are penalized by higher co-payments. Prescribing off-formulary drugs, if permitted at all, might require extensive additional and onerous paperwork by the physician and considerable cost to the patient. Adherence with the formulary list becomes the path of least resistance for physician and patient alike.

About the same time that managed care and fixed formularies came into existence, a proliferation of direct pharmaceutical advertising to consumers began. This direct-to-consumer (DTC) marketing, of course, creates demand and that demand gets transferred to the physician through the patient. The doctor becomes confronted with specific requests for specific medications, a relatively new phenomenon in medical practice.

The ability to market prescribed medications directly to the general public may seem obvious or even inevitable. In fact, it is rare. Only two countries in the world allow direct marketing of prescription medications: New Zealand and the United States. Why should this be the case? Why does virtually every other country ban direct marketing of prescription drugs and the U.S. does not? The answer is, of course, cost.

Publicity enhances demand and demand increases consumptions (and hopefully corporate profits). Per capita use of pharmaceuticals in the United States is almost $800 per person. In Great Britain it is only $300/person and in Denmark, it is only $200/person. Are the British and Danish sicker than Americans because of this reduced medication consumption? The answer is no! Life expectance in Great Britain and Denmark is the same as in the United States and their per capita health care costs are about half of ours.

Another phenomenon that has transformed the American legal drug market has been the proliferation of over-the-counter "food supplements." This might also seem inevitable or even beneficial, but it has not always been the case. Prior to the Hatch Act (Orin Hatch, a politician from Utah), supplements were controlled by the FDA and had to be proven both "safe and effective" by their manufacturers. This requirement created two problems for the supplement industry. First, the testing involved is complex, expensive and time consuming. Second, and more important, is that many of these products, if not most, are neither effective nor safe. In fact, many can be medically dangerous.

With the passage of the Hatch Act, previously regulated substances were reclassified as "food supplements" rather than as drugs. The onerous necessity of FDA control suddenly disappeared. What followed was a massive increase in the supplement industry, which just happened to be well represented in Senator Hatch's home state of Utah. DNA testing of some of these products has proven that many herbal supplements do not, in fact, contain any of the active ingredients. Others may contain useless or even dangerous substances, none of which are now regulated by the FDA.

Calls to eliminate direct-to-consumer advertising of prescription drugs and re-introduce FDA control of supplements have both been soundly rejected. The economic pressures have been overwhelming from the pharmaceutical and supplement industries, neither of which want to see an increase in regulation or a decrease in their profits.

Another interesting phenomenon has been the internationalization of mail order medications. Drugs, which cost hundreds of dollars in the U.S., may be sold for pennies on the dollar out of our borders and often with no prescription at all. Efforts to increase the availability of such mail order sources have also met with ferocious resistance. Issues of drug safety are often evoked, even when the same company using the same strict quality control standards as in the United States produces the medications. The motivation for the opposition may well be profit margins more than public safety.

While the wonders of the pharmaceutical industry have transformed medical outcomes, the same industries have and continue to influence the medical marketplace. Physicians are deluged with a constant stream of very affable, very competent pharmaceutical represents, often several from the same company. Gifts, free lunches and dinners for the physician and his or her staff, trips, honorariums for pseudo-research and focus groups all used to come in an endless and abundant stream.

Long overdue legislation stopped the flow of these excesses in the nineties, but there are always opportunities, both legal and illegal to benefit from the pharmaceutical largess. In the end, it requires a concerted effort by physicians, the public and the pharmaceutical industry to recognize that profits, while necessary, cannot be the only motivation for those interested in healthcare if we are to achieve reasonable outcomes for a reasonable price. Health is not a commodity like others things, and does not always respond to market pressures. In fact, where healthcare is concerned, it's not just business.

www.nihcr.org/Drug_Spending

http://www.ajhp.org/site/Projecting_future_drug_expenditures_2012.pdf

http://www.pbs.org/newshour/rundown/2012/10/health-costs-how-the-us-compares-with-other-countries.html

B. PRESCRIPTION PAINKILLERS IN AMERICA: WHAT A PAIN!

Americans love their pills. This includes pain medications, the use of which has risen steadily since 1999 (increasing 4 times) while deaths from overdoses have increased proportionally. Even within the United States, some places seem to be habitual over-consumers, with painkiller prescription three times higher in Florida (reporting the highest use) than in Illinois (reporting the lowest use.) Louisiana, while not among the highest states for prescription of painkillers (6.8 kg/10,000 population) was among the top ten for drug overdose death rates (15/100,000 population) in 2008. The problem, however, is not limited to prescription pain drugs for legitimate uses, but spills over into an epidemic of non-medical uses as well. In fact, 12 million Americans engaged in non-medical use of prescription painkillers in 2010, or one out of twenty people over 12 years of age.

If the consequences were trivial, it might be different, but such indiscriminate use of painkillers, especially for non-medical uses, results in 15,000 deaths a year (2009), 500,000 emergency room visits and $72.5 billion each year in medical costs. The phenomenon of overdosing with painkillers strikes certain groups disproportionately. Men die from overdoses more often than women, middle-aged adults overdose more than other age groups, Whites and Native Americans overdose more than other ethnic groups and rural Americans overdose more than twice as often as city dwellers. This is of particular importance, of course, to our rural Central Louisiana parishes.

The availability of painkillers has now reached epidemic proportions. "Pill mills," where doctors make easy fortunes by prescribing inappropriate quantities of pain medications to inappropriate clients, have proliferated across the United States, particularly in Florida. Although there are attempts to better track the use and abuse of painkillers, the creativity of the criminal element, notably among less-than-scrupulous physicians, results in constant stream of pain pills for recreational use.

What can you do as an individual? Use painkillers only as prescribed, do not share or sell them to others and always keep them locked up. Young people have "pill parties," where they bring assorted medications, notably painkillers, to a party and consume them by the handful along with immoderate amounts of alcohol. The results, of course, can be catastrophic.

Health care providers should use painkillers judiciously. Although it often takes more time to explain why addictive pain medications should not be used than to write a prescription, it does no good to add addiction to a patient's list of chronic medical problems. Prescriptions should be limited in time and quantity and habitual users should agree to regular drug testing. State governments can improve their prescription monitoring systems, and, with the cooperation of licensing boards such as the Louisiana State Board of Medical Examiners, identify and prosecute those who prescribe inappropriately. States can also make sure that there are adequate programs for substance abuse at the community level.

Pain medications can and do become true "pain killers," resulting in the death of those who use them. It is the responsibility of individuals, health care providers and governmental entities to cooperate in addressing this epidemic. If you have a problem with pain medication, call 1-800-662-HELP.

www.cdc.gov/homeandrecreationalsafety/rxbrief/

http://www2c.cdc.gov/podcasts/player.asp?f=8629113

C. APPROACHING THE "POST-ANTIBIOTIC ERA?"

Infectious diseases were once the leading killers of the world. In the U.S. in 1900, pneumonia, TB and infectious diarrheas were the first three causes of death. By 1997 and beyond, heart disease and cancer dominated, while pneumonia had dropped to a distant 6th place. Since penicillin was first introduced in 1943, the entire medical landscape shifted, with infectious diseases steadily retreating. The public has always felt reassured that the proliferation of new and improved products would keep pace with the rapid appearance of what scientist call "resistant" germs. What has followed has been a race between human ingenuity and microbial evolution, with the same holding true for viral, fungal, parasitic diseases and other organisms.

Many microbes (and other microscopic organisms) proliferate in astonishing numbers and with breath-taking rapidity. They respond to changes in their environment by eventually developing and even transferring genetic resistance to each and every antibiotic that is thrown their way. Penicillin-resistant *Staphylococcus* was already identified before the mass introduction of penicillin. As each new antibiotic hit the market (tetracycline, erythromycin, methicillin, gentamicin, vancomycin, imipenem, ceftazidime, levofloxin, and more recently linezolid, daptomycin and ceftaroline), some resistant organisms have developed.

It is now estimated by the CDC that antibiotic resistant organisms cause over 2 million illnesses and 23,000 deaths each year. The top five culprits by number of cases are Streptococcus *pneumonieae* (1,200,000), *Campylobacter* (310,000), *Neisseria gonorrhaeae* (246,000), *Salmonella* (100,000) and Methicillin-resistant *Staphylococcus aureus* (MRSA) (80,000). One particular organism, *Clostridium difficile*, proliferates when antibiotics are given for other reasons and causes 250,000 cases and 14,000 deaths although it is not itself antibiotic resistant yet. *C. difficile* alone results in over a billion dollars of excess medical costs a year.

While this counter-attack of bacterial resistance has been increasing, the number of new antibiotics introduced has been steadily dwindling.

From 1980-1984, around 18 new antibiotics were developed. By 1995-1999, this number had dropped to 11 and from 2010-2012, only one new antibiotic was developed and approved.

Beyond the growing problem of resistance, antibiotics themselves are not without side effects, which result in one out of five emergency room visits. This number is particularly true in children under the age of 18 for whom drug reactions to antibiotics are the most common cause of medication side effects.

There is no doubt that the overuse of antibiotics has contributed to the worsening of this national crisis. While prescription patterns vary widely, the states with the highest antibiotic prescriptions rates per capita include Louisiana, Mississippi, Alabama, Arkansas, Tennessee, Kentucky, Ohio and West Virginia. The lowest rates include the states of California, Oregon, Washington, Colorado, New Hampshire and Vermont.

Although preventive measures vary with the organism, some of the most troublesome organisms are often found within the hospital setting and include *C. difficile*, *Enterobacteriaceae*, *Acinetobacter*, resistant *Candida* (fungus), *Enteroccoccus*, *Pseudomonas aeruginosa*, and MRSA. Both healthcare providers and patients should follow some simple (and not so simple) rules. For the public, wash your hands, long and hard, and take antibiotics only when needed and then only as directed. For providers, know the resistant organisms in your institutions. If you have drug-resistant organisms, personnel, especially the infection control practitioner, should be alerted within your own and other facilities. Staff and other patients should be protected from infectious cases and all external medical devices (including catheters, IV lines, ventilators and drains) should be removed as soon as possible.

The CDC offers a 4-part solution to tackling this vexing problem: (1) Prevent infections, (2) Track resistance patterns, (3) Practice antibiotic stewardship and (4) Develop new antibiotics and diagnostic tests. Antibiotics are wonderful tools, but they are double-edged swords if not used correctly. If you do not need antibiotics, do not insist on getting them. Remember, it takes a busy doctor a couple of minutes to write a prescription, but 20 or more to explain why they should not be prescribed because you are your loved will not benefit. If we do not use antibiotics wisely, we may well enter into the "post antibiotic era" when none are available.

http://www.cdc.gov/drugresistance/threat-report-2013

D. DYING TO BE YOUNG AND POTENT

Aging carries with it a host of medical issues for men, among them a gradual reduction in testosterone levels. One of the many consequences of this reduction may be erectile dysfunction ("ED"). It is estimated that around 5% of 40-year old men and up to 25% of 65 year-old men suffer from erectile dysfunction. A normal man can fail to achieve an erection 20% of the time, but it should not happen over 50% of the time. Fatigue, stress, excess alcohol, arteriosclerosis, hypertension, diabetes, many medications and other common factors can cause erectile dysfunction. The estimated 5 million men in the U.S. suffering from low testosterone represent an irresistible and lucrative market.

Legitimate concerns about potency, coupled with anxieties associated with aging of the baby boomers, has spawned a multi-billion dollar industry for the treatment of erectile dysfunction. Sales of Viagra and Cialis exceed one billion dollars each. The top 100 most-prescribed medications include Viagra (18th), Cialis (21st) and Levitra (96th), all three medications for erectile dysfunction, with total prescriptions of the three exceeding 16 million a year.

Testosterone replacement in gels, patches and injections, all used for decreased potency associated with "Low T", has now reached sales of 1.6 billion a year. Androgel brought in 1.14 billion in sales in 2013 and Axiron resulted in 168 million in sales (an 85% increase from 2011). Heavy direct-to-consumer (DTC) advertising by pharmaceutical firms has helped boost sales of all such medications significantly, a well-documented phenomena. In fact, sales of testosterone have increased five times from 2000 to 2011, now reaching 5.3 million prescriptions a year. What older man doesn't want to feel a newfound surge of energy, stamina and sexual potency?

Like all medications, however, there is no such thing as a free lunch. While testosterone does increase muscle mass and physical stamina, there is also evidence that it worsens benign prostatic hypertrophy (enlargement of the prostate) and aggravates prostate cancer, both contraindications to its use. What is less well known is that it may also increase rates of heart attacks. A New England Journal of

Medicine study in 2010 reported that testosterone replacement caused a significant increase in cardiac risk. Another more recent study of over 8,000 men by the U.S. Veteran's Administration, published in the Journal of the American Medical Association (JAMA), confirmed a 29% increase in the risk of having a heart attack in the testosterone replacement group. In that particular elderly population, however, it should be mentioned that many of the men had underlying heart disease or diabetes.

Associate editors for the JAMA, Anne Cappola, was quoted by Nicole Ostrow at Bloomberg News as saying that some "think it's the fountain of youth. It's going to give them back sexual performance, strength and endurance. The direct marketing of testosterone is playing into that. There needs to be that other voice saying there's no medication out there with all benefit and no risk. There's always a tradeoff."

As distressing as aging is, especially to those of the baby boomer generation, a decrease in sexual potency may be one of the prices to be paid for longevity. Trying to achieve sexual performance through pills, patches and gels may be increasing cardiac risk for debatable benefits. Those anxious to sell us the "fountain of youth" need to make it clear that there is always a risk/benefit ratio with all drugs and those risks should never exceed the real or imagined benefits they confer.

Basaria, Shehzad et al. "Adverse Events Associated with Testosterone Administration," N Engl J Med 2010; 363:109-122.

www.bloomberg.com/news/2013-11-05/testosterone-drugs-raise-heart-risk-in-1-billion-market.html

Vigen, R. et al. "Association of Testosterone Therapy with Mortality, Myocardial Infarction, and Stroke in Men with Low Testosterone Levels," JAMA 2013;310(17) 1829-1836.

E. IMMUNIZATIONS: NOT JUST FOR KIDS

Pediatricians have become very adept at the use of LINKS (Louisiana Immunization Network for Kids Statewide), an electronic tracking system for vaccinations introduced through the Louisiana Office of Public Health. The system is so successful that it has resulted in national recognition as well as vaccination rates in Louisiana that largely exceed national averages. (Louisiana was 25/50 states in America's Health Rankings for children and 6/50 for adolescents, 2013.)

What is not as well known is that there are a half-a-dozen other immunizations that are recommended for adult. Although LINKS can be used for adult vaccinations, it has not been used extensively in that way because of the intermittent nature and lower volumes inherent in adult vaccinations. There is also a lack of familiarity by some providers although the push toward meaningful use of electronic health records may provide a certain incentive.

Influenza remains the most obvious and well-recognized adult vaccination. The CDC has increased recommendations for flu vaccine to now include almost everyone older than 6 months of age. The flu virus has the ability to change its genetic makeup and undergo what is called antigenic shift and drift. This means that a new vaccine must be developed each year based on the best educated guesses and data from flu surveillance sites all over the world. Because flu vaccines have to be formulated every year, receiving a new flu shot should be an annual ritual. Even though seasonal flu season peaks in February, adults (and children) should be vaccinated as early as September and extending through March.

Although most people know that their "tetanus shot" (actually tetanus/diphtheria or TD) needs to be updated every ten years, remembering your last shot date becomes a mnemonic challenge. Being registered in the LINKS system through the health unit or your physician's office can jog your memory. But what is less well known is that at least one booster needs to be with Tdap (tetanus, diphtheria and pertussis or whooping cough) and not tetanus alone. The reason is that the body's immunity to pertussis tends to wane with time. Pertussis (whooping cough) can manifest itself in adults as a chronic, annoying cough, unlike the life threatening form in young children. Parents or grandparents can inadvertently transmit pertussis to their infant children or grandchildren who might be incompletely vaccinated.

Another "adult" vaccine is the HPV or Human Papilloma Virus. This particular vaccine protects against cervical cancer as well as most forms of oral cancers and genital warts. It should be administered as early as 11 years old and should be completed prior to becoming sexually active. It can, however, be safely administered up to 26 years of age in women and 21 years of age in men. Three doses are required and cost remains an issue in some cases since it can be $120/HPV vaccination.

The Herpes Zoster vaccine is an adult vaccine that is recommended after 60 years of age (although it can be given as early as 50). It prevents or shortens outbreaks of shingles, related to reactivation of the varicella virus (chicken pox). While not usually life threatening, shingles can be a painful and debilitating experience. Vaccine cost might be a factor when it is not covered by insurance since it costs around $250.

Another geriatric immunization is the pneumococcal vaccine, or the so-called "pneumonia shot." The polysaccharide form is indicated in adults over 65 years of age as well as some susceptible individuals prior to that time. It protects against pneumococcal pneumonia, a common cause of illness or death in the elderly.

In short, immunizations do not stop after childhood. Influenza, Tdap, HPV, Zoster and Pneumococcal are five that should be administered to adults. Others, such as MMR (Measles, mumps, and rubella) or Hepatitis A may be required under certain circumstances, especially if vaccination documentation is limited or foreign travel expected. In case of doubt, check with your physician, the Office of Public Health, or CDC.gov for more information.

www.cdc.gov/vaccines/

www.americashealthrankings.org

http://www.cdc.gov/vaccines/schedules/easy-to-read/adult.html

F. ROBOTIC SURGERY:
DISSECTING HYPE FROM REALITY

Everyone has heard of one of the latest technological advances, robotic surgery. Developed in the 1980's and approved in the 90's, robotic surgery swept across the United States and had been adopted by over a fourth of hospitals by 2011. In 2012, over 367,000 robotic surgeries were performed in the United States, including prostatectomies, hysterectomies, nephrectomies, cholecystectomies, gastric by-pass surgeries, heart valve repairs and many other procedures. This was a 26% increase over the number performed a year earlier, a clear indication of rapid technological adoption.

Although supporters insist on the quicker recovery times, reduced pain and blood loss compared to traditional "open" surgeries, there remains uncertainty about the advantages over non-robotic assisted laparoscopic surgery where that is an option. What is certain is that robotic surgery adds to the cost of surgery. Use of a robot in any procedure added around 13% (or $3,200) to the cost of a procedure in 2007 (New England Journal of Medicine, 2010). The cost of the machine alone is around $2.0 million, with service contracts over $150,000/year and disposable instruments kits costing up $1,000 each (and sometimes requiring up to half a dozen or more per surgery.)

The controversy is particularly heated with respect to hysterectomies. While use of a robot may not decrease complications, it clearly increases cost when robotic hysterectomies ($8,868) are compared with laparoscopic hysterectomies ($6,679). This has led to the American Congress of Obstetricians and Gynecologists to release a statement that there is "no good data proving that robotic hysterectomy is even as good as, let along better, than existing, far less costly, minimally invasive alternatives." (in this case they were referring to trans-vaginal non-robotic laparoscopic hysterectomy.)

Other procedures, whether they are prostatectomies, mitral-valve repairs, cholecystectomies or gastric by-pass, all add significant cost when performed with robotic assistance. Even when the procedures are not reimbursed at a higher rate than traditional procedures, hospitals appear to be willing to absorb the cost differential for whatever reason. This may be from perceived quality to one of many examples of what is sometimes called the "technology *du jour*" or the latest, shiniest tool in the toolbox (often used for marketing purposes.)

All innovative technologies and new medications undergo what is known as a "phase of enthusiasm" during which early adopters embrace the new product or technology and proclaim its superiority. What inevitably follows is the "phase of deception" during which complications, side effects and cost considerations become apparent. Usage may decline, but will only disappear if the new product completely fails to live up to its expectations or its cost clearly exceeds its benefit. In most cases, the product or technology plateaus out at a level commensurate with its true medical value to society.

This whole notion of value remains critical, since value is determined by quality divided by cost. If the cost is prohibitive, the quality may be enhanced, but the value to the society and to the individual drops. Those cost increases, despite quality, can become so high that there is a point of diminishing returns. Small increases in quality can become so costly that they are simply not worth it. It remains to be seen whether robotic surgery is here to stay and, if so, for what indications. Robotic technologies are surely here to stay, with progressive improvements in hardware and software sophistication. That being said, it is always desirable to separate hype and marketing from the true value of any product or procedure.

Questions Arise about Robotic Surgery's Cost, Effectiveness. Medscape. Apr 23, 2013.

http://www.medscape.com/viewarticle/802971

Is Robotic Surgery Worth It's Price? Medscape. Jun 20, 2013.

http://www.medscape.com/viewarticle/806484

Barbash, GI and Glied, SA. "New Technology and Health Care Costs—The Case of Robot-Assisted Surgery." N Engl J Med 2010;363: 701-704.

G. STATINS AND MEMORY LOSS: UNWARRENTED CONTROVERSY

In February 2012, the FDA added a warning on statins that they could possibly cause minor and reversible (or irreversible) cognitive side effects in some individuals. This news, of course, resulted in waves of consternation among some of the 20 million Americans, many of them elderly, who currently take some form of statin to lower their cholesterol. What is the controversy and what are the implications for patients and providers?

Statins are HMG-CoA reductase inhibitors, which block an enzyme responsible for the production of cholesterol. They have demonstrated their effectiveness over the years by reducing cardiovascular morbidity and mortality up to 40-50%, a dramatic and positive development. They have been so successful that some experts have suggested in a tongue-in-cheek manner that they should be "put in the water supply." They have also been highly profitable to the pharmaceutical industry with $130 billion dollars in cumulative sales for atorvastatin (Lipitor) alone.

Several large studies (HPS or Heart Protection Study and PROSPER or Prospective Study of Pravastatin in the Elderly at Risk) did address cognitive issues among others. They concluded that there was no evidence of memory decline in the patients in the study. In fact, other studies concluded there might be a slight delay in the development of Alzheimer's disease and a possible improvement in memory in those who take statins.

Why then the recent FDA warning? All medications have idiosyncratic effects. There is "no such thing as a free lunch," or, in medical terms, there is always a risk-benefit ratio with all medications. The FDA receives reports from physicians through a surveillance system called MedWatch. Because of the huge number of individual receiving statins, some of these people experienced various degrees of reversible or irreversible memory loss. These reports, unlike scientific studies, are not standardized or double-blinded. It is impossible to verify the validity of the observations, which are rarely associated with objective studies.

Although this memory effect seems to be excessively rare, and possibly reversible with cessation of the drug or changing to a different statin, it still seemed appropriate to include the warning in the official FDA sanctioned product warnings. (The same holds true for the possibility of an increase in blood sugar levels, which may be associated with statin use as well.)

Since statins have been so successful and so widely prescribed, any publicity related to their possible unfavorable effects is sure to get wide coverage. On the one hand, the popular press thrives on the fear factor. On the other hand, long-term health benefits, while important to public health, may not be considered newsworthy. The bottom line is that the worries about statin-related memory loss appear to be minimal, while the tremendous positive effects are indisputable.

If you experience memory loss with any statin (or any other medication), be sure to let your doctor know. There are appropriate standardized tests, some simple and some more complex, to evaluate memory loss. Reducing cholesterol, safely and effectively, has been one of the triumphs of modern medicine (along with reductions and blood pressure). Don't let unreasonable anxiety stop you from doing the right thing for your long-term health.

Wagstaff, LR et al., "Statin-Associated Memory Loss: Analysis of 60 Case Reports and Review of the Literature." Pharmacotherapy. 2003;(23)(7)

H. "BATH SALTS," "SYNTHETIC COCAINE" OR 3, 4-METHYLENEDIOXYPYROVALERONE (MDPV)

Backyard chemists are constantly looking for new and creative substances that are still legal, stimulating and provide hefty profits. One of the latest was 3,4-Methylenedioxypyrovalerone (MDPV) and a series of closely related chemical substances. MDPV has an amphetamine-like effect, which lasts several hours, followed by prolonged after-effects lasting several hours or days and sometimes associated with suicidal ideation.

This substance was most often sold as so-called "bath salts" under the brand names of Ivory Wave, Ocean, Charge +, White Lightening, Scarface, Hurricane Charlie, Red Dove, Cloud 9, White Dove and many others. The brightly colored packages contained less than a gram of product and were clearly marked "Not for Human Consumption," an obvious example of false and deceptive advertising. The locations of sales (tobacco shops and convenience stores) are not the usual venues for traditional "bath salts," especially in quantities totally inadequate for a normal bath. It is also sold on-line as "M.D.P.V. Garden Insect Deterrent," "pH Optimizer" or even "Plant Food." Prices range from $30 a gram to as much as $170 a gram, with individual doses ranging from 200 to 500 mg/package. In contrast, true "bath salts" (used in bath water) cost a few pennies a gram and are sold in much larger quantities.

These products are being snorted or swallowed. They can also be sprayed on dried plants of various sorts and smoked. Regardless of the route of ingestions, the effects include a mild sense of euphoria and stimulation, accompanied by insomnia, anxiety, depression, hyperactivity, hallucinations and an increased heart rate. Although the initial effects wear off in a couple of hours, the user may have longer lasting feelings of depression, anxiety, sleep disturbance and paranoia. Some users end up in the emergency room and those cases are subsequently reported to the Louisiana Poison Center. Of the 253 cases reported to ERs nationwide (as of Jan. 2, 2011), 158 cases (or

62%) came from Louisiana. For some unknown reason, Louisiana became a national testing site for such products before their subsequent widespread distribution around the United States.

Although mortality and true addiction appear limited, the potential for serious medical consequences exists. Some states, including Louisiana, began outlawing MDPV early in 2011 and the federal government subsequently took action in September 7, 2011. The DEA designated MDPV and its derivatives as Class 1 controlled substances, making them illegal to possess, a temporary solution that lasted only a year. But creative and unscrupulous chemists seem to be working faster than legislators and various other dangerous substances proliferate as soon as one has been identified and outlawed.

Another class of recreations drugs is "synthetic marijuana," a group of substances chemically related to the active ingredient of real marijuana. These substances are soaked with or sprayed on tobacco and often sold under the label of "Spice" or "K2." Once again, many chemical variants of these substances are possible and law enforcement remains one step behind creative chemists, both professionals and amateurs.

One of the latest kids on the block, but surely not the last, appears to be phenazepam, a depressant sold as an "air freshener" and apparently manufactured in Russia. The same country appears to be the origin of an injectable product, "krocodil," which can cause the flesh to rot off in a massive debilitating necrosis. Although both can be added to the list of Schedule 1 drugs, making them susceptible to seizure, it still takes time to get such proposals through the legislative process. An alternative is to have the Secretary of the Louisiana Department of Health and Hospitals declare them (or other designer drugs) as hazardous. As such, they can be pulled off the shelves (if they are being sold in convenience stores or head shops) and held as contraband until they can be legitimately added to definitive legislation. Such an expedited declaration allows removal of dangerous substances quickly pending other more time consuming official procedures. If a substance proves to be truly innocuous, it can always be returned to the supplier.

Although it may be impossible to remove all substances susceptible to abuse from those determined to use them, obvious examples of documented dangerous substances should be removed from legal sale as was done with MDPV. The prompt actions taken against "Bath Salts" and "Synthetic Marijuana" demonstrated that local health officials and state and federal government agencies can work together quickly and efficiently to remove at least one set of dangerous substances from the hands of consumers. Addition of further legal tools will help us remain one step of the backyard chemists both here and abroad. We may not be able to save all people from their self-destructive tendencies, but we can make it harder for them to indulge.

Bath Salts and Synthetic Cannabinoids: A Review. Medscape. Mar 01, 2012.

http://www.medscape.com/viewarticle/765892

http://en.wikipedia.org/wiki/Designer_drug

I. CHOOSING WISELY: THE AMERICAN BOARD OF INTERNAL MEDICINE'S RECOMMENDATIONS FOR TESTS AND PROCEDURES NOT TO HAVE DONE!

In this era of high-tech medicine, there are a plethora of wonderful tests and procedures that your doctor can order. Although it may seem intuitive that the "more the better," that is not always the case. Some tests may actually be dangerous and many are very expensive. Each time doctors order a test, the question should always be "do the benefits of the information exceed the risks" (and the costs.) Since we are currently spending over 2.7 trillion dollars a year (over 16% of the gross domestic product) on medical care, the burden of medical costs is crowding out other expenditures and making the nation less competitive in the world market. In addition, over 225,000 deaths a year are considered "iatrogenic" (related to medical care) and it is estimated that less than 20% of such cases are reported.

The American Board of Internal Medicine (ABIM) asked doctors in various fields to list 5 tests that they felt should NOT be done, since their cost (or risks) exceeded the expected benefits. Although some of the tests and procedures are uncommon, many are very common and often considered "indispensable." Following are a few of the selections from this list of things not to be done from three of the leading medical organizations.

The American College of Physicians (ACP) does NOT recommend getting EKGs in individuals without symptoms and with low cardiac risk. They do NOT recommend getting x-ray studies of the back in patients with non-specific back pain of short duration (and without neurological symptoms). The ACP does NOT recommend chest x-rays in patients prior to surgery when there is no suspicion of thoracic problems.

The American Academy of Family Physicians (AAFP) does NOT recommend antibiotics for the treatment of sinusitis lasting less than seven days. They do NOT recommend DEXA (bone density) screening in women less than 65 or men less than 70 without known risk factors. The AAFP (and others) do not recommend Pap smears in women younger than 21 or women older than 65 with a normal prior test, or any woman after a hysterectomy. The same group does NOT recommend induced labor or Cesarean sections prior to 39 weeks gestation without documented true medical indications. The AAFP does NOT recommend screening carotid ultrasounds (looking for blockage in the arteries of the neck) in adults without symptoms.

The American Academy of Pediatrics (AAP) does NOT recommend antibiotics for viral respiratory illnesses in children. They do NOT recommend cough and cold medicines for children under four years of age. The AAP does not recommend a CT (or MRI) of the head for children with simple febrile (related to fever) seizures. Similarly, they do NOT recommend abdominal CTs for the routine evaluation of abdominal pain.

There are many more recommendations of tests NOT to perform listed under the ABIM "Choosing Wisely" list. Before the uncertainty of medical situations and the constant dread of litigation, the tendency has been to perform tests that may not really be medically indicated. The current program gives solid scientific justifications for these decisions to abstain from unnecessary testing. Sometimes more is not better and, as always, the physicians' mantra should be *primum non nocere*" (first, do no harm), whether it be to the patient or the national debt.

www.choosingwisely.org/doctor-patient-lists

J. ELECTRONIC HEALTH RECORDS: COMING TO A MEDICAL PROVIDER NEAR YOU!

The electronic revolution has slowly but surely begun to filter down to the physician level in Louisiana as elsewhere in the U.S. As with most technological advances, there are early adopters and late adopters. That Electronic Health Records (EHRs) are here to stay, however, is inevitable.

The American Recovery and Reinvestment Act (ARRA) of 2009 contained significant health information technology grants designed to increase the use of EHRs and achieve "meaningful use." The five priorities of "meaningful use" are: (1) Improving safety, quality and efficiency while reducing health disparities, (2) Engaging patients and families in their own care, (3) Improving care coordination, (4) Improving population and public health and (5) Ensuring privacy and security of personal health information (PHI).

Significant financial incentives are in place for practitioners accepting Medicaid (practices with over 30% Medicaid patients) and non-hospital based Medicare. The former can receive up to $63,750 in incentives and the latter can receive up to $44,000 over five years. The plan for implantation is staged and the first incentives could be received for just buying an EHR system. Progressively, however, the practitioner must demonstrate that they are achieving "meaningful use" to obtain subsequent incentives, which phase out entirely in 2016 for Medicare.

"Meaningful use" entails achieving objectives in a series of "core requirements" (15) and "menu set" objectives (5). The former include such standard information as allergies, demographic information, problem and medication lists, vital signs, smoking status and other objectives. While the "menu set" includes such objectives as drug formulary checks, patient education resources, immunization records, patient reminders and others.

There are also "Clinical Quality Measures" currently relating to hypertension, tobacco use and weight that must be incorporated in 2011 and 2012. These will be followed by measures of breast and colorectal cancer screening, monitoring of glycosylated hemoglobin values (for diabetics) and tobacco cessation.

The AARA legislation contains both the carrots of paid incentives and the sticks of reduced reimbursements and incentives over time to encourage physicians to get on the EHR bandwagon. The Louisiana Health Information Technology (LHIT) Resource Center was established to assist 1,400 priority primary care providers to achieve meaningful use criteria. It is hoped that all Americans will have access to EHRs by 2014, although this may be an unrealistic expectation.

Ultimately, it is hoped that all providers will also be hooked up to Health Information Exchanges, which will allow transmission of health information between various providers (including hospitals and outpatient clinicians.) The goal is to achieve coordination of care and reduce some of the horrendous waste in duplication of services and fragmented care.

Implementation of EHRs has been spotty for a number of reasons. Inertia tends to block some innovations, while expense and drops of productivity among providers are other problems. Even though EHRs are supposed to achieve cost savings for both the provider and patients, they are sometimes difficult to substantiate in the painful initial period of implementation. To add to the confusion, there are multiple vendors of multiple systems and providers are hesitant to make the considerable investment of time and resources without substantial reassurances of success. That, in fact, is the point of the initial financial incentives.

So prepare for your provider to have a tablet or a laptop, with or without a stethoscope, when you see him or her at your next appointment. For some patients, this has already occurred. For others it will be a disconcerting shock. Whatever your reaction, this "Brave New World" of Electronic Health Records is here to stay.

http://lhcqf.org/lhit-about

http://www.nytimes.com/2012/10/09/health/the-ups-and-downs-of-electronic-medical-records-the-digital-doctor.html?pagewanted=all&_r=0

http://www.cms.gov/Regulations-and-Guidance/Legislation/EHRIncentivePrograms/index.html

CHAPTER VI
CREEPY CRAWLERS
(AND FLYERS, TOO)

A. BEDBUGS: THEY'RE BACK!

Bedbugs (*Cimex lectularius*) have long been the scourges of the traveler. Almost eliminated after World War II with the extensive use of DDT, they have come back with a vengeance worldwide. Although they do not transmit human illnesses, they feed off human blood and cause irritating bites that can swell up in sensitive individuals. They are also notoriously secretive and can hide out during the day in the tiniest nooks and crevices in mattresses, furniture and wallpaper making them difficult to identify and eradicate.

The adults are small (about ¼ inch), flat and somewhat ovoid in shape. They are brown or reddish brown, depending on whether they have ingested blood. An adult female can lay 2 or 3 eggs per day and up to 200 or more in their lifetime. The eggs hatch in about nine days and go through five nymph stages (lasting 10 days or more) before reaching adulthood. Each stage requires a blood meal for further development. Adults can survive months without feeding. They do not travel great distances, but can hitchhike in clothes, luggage, furniture or other items.

Eliminating them proves a huge challenge. Multiple pesticide agents are available, including agents for cracks and crevices, indoor surfaces and indoor spaces. Agents for cracks and crevices are generally dusts or sprays. Indoor surface treatments include residual sprays or dusts, while indoor space treatments are contact aerosols. Some of the available products cannot be used on mattresses due to concerns of neurotoxicity and manufacturer's recommendations should be strictly observed. There is controversy about the use of foggers, since some professionals feel that they force the insects into more inaccessible locations from which they emerge later. Heating the room to 113 degrees Fahrenheit (45 degrees Celsius) can also kill the bugs, but is cumbersome and expensive. Steam treating rugs and drapes, replacement of mattresses and furniture, and sealing of all cracks and crevices should be implemented.

How do you protect yourself? First, inspect the edges of all mattresses, even in luxury hotels, for the presence of telltale black spots around the mattress seams. These spots are bedbug's fecal matter. Second, since bedbugs hide in loose wallpaper and in other cracks and crevices, do not stay in a room that has obvious evidence of poor maintenance. Third, do not leave your luggage on the floor and keep it closed when possible. Although bedbugs may hitchhike in your luggage, they usually do not stay on a moving person. Fourth, there are portable sprays for travelers to use. And fifth, when you return, be sure to wash your clothes in hot water and inspect and vacuum your luggage to make sure you don't have any unwanted hitchhikers.

Given the elusive nature of the bugs, their nocturnal nature, and their prolonged survival without blood meals, they have quickly become the scourge of the traveler and the innkeeper. With worldwide travel, the potential for infestation in even the smallest communities only becomes a question of time. Eradication of these pests in the home or business usually requires professional assistance. Even then, the development of resistance in bedbugs to some of the routine pesticides makes the job of eradication more and more difficult. So when you travel, follow the advice above and remember, sleep tight and don't let the bedbugs bite.

http://www.cdc.gov/parasites/bedbugs/

B. OF LICE AND MEN

Head lice, *Pediculus humanus capitis*, are every parent's nightmare. These nasty little creatures live near the scalp and feed on human blood. They lay eggs (nits), which appear as tiny white spots, generally ¼ inch from the scalp attached to individual strands of hair. Although they cannot jump or fly, lice are easily transmitted from head to head by contact. Rarely, they can be transmitted by contact with infected pillows, scarves, other clothing or personal items such as combs.

The good news is that head lice do not transmit any more serious diseases. They do, however, cause irritation of the scalp, intense itching (especially at night) and cause considerable disruption if the school happens to enforce a "No nit" policy (when children cannot return to school if any nits are still present.)

It is estimated that there are around 10 million cases every year in the United States, mostly in children from 3 to 11 years old. It affects Caucasians more than Afro-Americans because of the predilection of lice for straighter, larger diameter hair for which they are better adapted.

If your child is diagnosed, it is important to check all family members, especially other children. There are several over-the-counter treatments (Pyrethrin or Permethrin lotions). Strict adherence to product recommendations is necessary since some over-the-counter agents are not approved for children less than 2 years of age. These products kill the adult lice, but not the eggs (nits). Nit removal with special combs is also recommended. It is always necessary to re-treat, usually in 9-10 days, in order to kill any lice that may have hatched from remaining eggs. Bedding and clothing should also be machine washed and dried. Combs should be soaked in hot water (130 F or higher) for 10 minutes and floors and carpets should be vacuumed to remove hair.

A couple of re-treatments with over-the-counter products may be necessary. Unfortunately, some lice are resistant to these products and require use of prescription medications such as Malathion or Lindane. These organo-chloride products kill the hatched lice, but are only partially effective against the eggs. They, like the other agents, require re-treatment in 7-9 days. They are both trickier to use and can cause more significant topical irritation. Strict adherence to manufacturer's recommendations is imperative since there are specific age and weight requirements.

The CDC does not recommend "No-nit" policies. Once a child is treated for the first time, they should be able to return to school. Head lice are common and not a source of other transmissible diseases. Parents should be reassured that lice are not an indication of personal cleanliness, but a common nuisance that can affect both kings and paupers.

www.cdc.gov/parasites/lice/

C. SCABIES: THE BURROWING MIGHTY MITE

Scabies, *Sarcoptes scabiei var. hominis*, continues to plague mankind despite our best attempts to eradicate it. The creatures, small mites related to spiders, have eight legs in their adult form and live off flakes of dead skin. People become infected when a gravid (pregnant) female passes from person to person after direct, prolonged, skin-to-skin contact. That female digs into the skin to form a "permanent" burrow and lays eggs that hatch in 3-5 days as nymphs. The nymphs locate their own "molting pouches," where they undergo several transformations into an adult males and females. Adult mites then mate and the females go off to establish new "permanent" burrows.

Because it takes some time to complete the cycle and develop a sufficient adult population, symptoms may begin 2-6 weeks after exposure. The infected host reacts to the presence of the burrowing adults with a local allergic reaction, resulting in intense itching, often worse at night. Sites of infestation include the wrists, elbows, armpits, hands, waistline, buttocks and external genitalia. Because of this latter predilection, scabies is often included as a sexually transmitted disease.

Usually there are only 10-15 adult mites on a normal host, but when scabies occurs on someone who is profoundly immune-compromised (very low immunity, such as with the use of steroids, chemotherapy, uncontrolled AIDS or bad diabetes), there may be thousands or millions of mites. This results in unsightly thick layers of skin or "Crusted Scabies or Norwegian Scabies," which is highly contagious to family and caregivers given the enormous number of organisms.

Scabies is usually relatively easy to treat with topical products such as Permethrin Cream (*Elimite*) or Crotamiton lotion or cream. When itching continues over 2-4 weeks in normal individuals, a second application may be necessary. Lindane lotion is sometimes used in difficult cases, although it can be neurotoxic in children. Ivermectin, an oral agent, is occasionally required in cases of unresponsive "Crusted Scabies," where millions of mites may be present.

Since the mites can only live 2-3 days off a person, the environment does not remain infectious. Washing clothing and sheets in hot water and drying in a hot dryer kills the organisms because mites are very sensitive to heat and will die at 122 degrees Fahrenheit or higher. Although animals can get scabies, they have their own species and human scabies does not infect animals or vice versa.

Once treatment is begun, the infected individual should be able to return to work the next day. If they were symptomatic with itching, especially between the fingers, then gloves should be used for a few days. Family members should be treated because of the possibility of prolonged skin-to-skin contact, but healthcare co-workers do not need to be treated if contact has only been casual.

The exception is for "Crusted Scabies," where the numbers of mites is so large that contagion is very likely. Affected individuals must be isolated and all contacts (and their families) should be aggressively treated. Such cases are the exception and not the rule. Prior to effective treatments, scabies infestations tormented those infested as well as their entire extended family. Today, a simple application (or two) of permethrin cream will clear up this pesky acarian, which nonetheless remains a constant, if unwanted, human companion.

www.cdc.gov/parasites/scabies/

D. FORMOSAN TERMITES: AN UNWANTED ASIAN INVADER

Formosan termites, *Coptotermes formosanus* Sharaki, are one of the several subterranean termites that now exist in Louisiana. The indigenous species are smaller, less aggressive and form smaller colonies than their Asian cousins. In fact, Formosan termites actually came from Southern China, not Formosa (the island of Taiwan), in 1945 when military materials on palettes of infested wood, were repatriated from the Far East. These contaminated articles came through one of several naval bases in New Orleans, where the termites found a warm and welcoming climate.

After proliferating for over two decades, they were identified in 1966 after they had firmly established themselves in Orleans and Calcasieu Parishes. By 2001, they were found in most South Louisiana parishes as well as St. Landry and Sabine Parishes to the north. By 2008, they were located in Vernon, Concordia, Rapides and Avoyelles Parish in Central Louisiana. Natchitoches Parish fell to their insatiable jaws in 2009. It is assumed that they are currently located in all 64 Louisiana parishes, but have not yet been formally identified.

Formosan termites form very large colonies, containing from 500,000 to over 2,000,000 insects. Each colony contains a king and queen that can lay over 1,000 eggs a day. Eggs develop into larval forms which can differentiate into workers, soldiers or alates (winged versions that fly off to mate and establish new colonies, after which they remove their own wings.)

Colonies must have contact with moist soil as a source of water. Workers, who are constantly foraging for new sources of food in the form of wood or other sources of cellulose, can construct burrows that lead from the ground up brick or cement pillars to wood beams above the soil. Exceptionally, a colony may be established above ground in a location with constantly wet wood, such as rafters under a roof leak, and form an "aerial nest."

Formosan termites are voracious and aggressive. Soldiers secrete a poison from their hard, tear-shaped heads, armed with sharp mandibles, that kills their enemies, including gentler native termite species. Alates (the flying versions) can be seen congregating around light sources at night when they swarm, something that differentiates them from their diurnal native cousins.

Since all termites are attracted to wood, it is advisable to avoid railroad ties and even mulch for landscaping in warm, Southern climates. Potted plants, shrubs and trees should be kept away from close contact with your home and always leave enough space for proper visibility for regular termite inspections. Liquid termiticides exist in either repellant or contact forms. Contact termiticides need to form a continuous barrier and a gap as small as $1/16^{th}$ of an inch can provide access for termites to a previously protected zone. In addition, any disruption of the soil where a contact termiticide has been applied will neutralize the effect by creating gaps.

The choice of control will be a function of construction type, proper application and whether it is for eradication of a current infestation or prevention of future infestations. Under any circumstances, always avoid wood to soil contact, especially in our moist climate, so perfect for this unwanted "Formosan" invader.

(Thanks to Carrie Owen of the ID-EPI Department of the Louisiana Office of Public Health for her inspiration.)

http://www.ars.usda.gov/is/ar/archive/oct98/term1098.htm

E. HONEY, CURE FOR HAY FEVER: WIVE'S TALE OR FACT?

Seasonal allergies (seasonal allergic rhinitis or "hay fever") affect over 36 million Americans each year. When the flowers and trees begin to bloom and the pollen fills the air, many people develop the usual symptoms of a runny nose, sneezing, coughing and red, watery eyes. Although it can just be a mild nuisance, the symptoms can be so severe that it results in a loss of work or school time.

The length and timing of the problem depends on what triggers the allergies. Seasonal allergic rhinitis (as opposed to year around perennial allergies) has many possible suspects, including trees, flowering shrubs, grasses and many more pollen producing plants. Some people have more symptoms in the spring, while others suffer more in the fall, depending on the particular agents.

Pollen acts as an allergen and stimulates the body to produce special white cells (Helper Type 2 T cells), which in turn activate eosinophil and antibody (IgE) production. With repeated exposures, most people will "down regulate" this system with production of other specialized white cells (Helper Type 1 T cells). For unknown reasons, some people do not benefit from this down regulation in childhood and allergic symptoms remain acute during adulthood. When allergens (pollen) react with the IgE antibody, they provoke the release of histamine from special cells (mast cells), which in turn results in tissue swelling and redness. In the case of allergic rhinitis, the reactions are mostly limited to the mucous membranes of the nose and eyes, but may affect the upper airways. In short, the person suffers from unpleasant symptoms as long as pollen (or other allergens) is around.

So what can be done? Reducing the exposure to pollen provides some relief, so staying indoors can help. Many people use oral antihistamines to blunt the allergic response. Some such agents are available over the counter and include cetirizine, desloratadine, and loratadine. Although they are "non-sedating," some patients still suffer from daytime sleepiness with these products. Other choices include topical nasal steroids such as beclomethasone, flunisolide, fluticasone and triamcinalone spays, which should be used daily during peak pollen season. Many people also use the topical vasoconstrictor, Afrin or the generic equivalent, but they simply reduce swelling and do not address the underlying allergic problem. In addition, long term Afrin or other vasoconstrictor use can result in aggravation of symptoms. In severe allergic cases, patients can undergo desensitization shots that alter the body's response to specific allergens (pollen or others.)

That brings us to honey. There are anecdotal reports that use of locally made honey reduces seasonal rhinitis symptoms. According to speculation, the local pollen contained in the honey results in desensitization of the host because of continued small exposures to local pollen allergens. The usual accepted dose of honey appears to be two teaspoons a day during the pollen season. A small, unpublished study at Xavier University suggested that those using local versus non-local honey had an improvement in their symptoms. Since the honey treatment is not expensive or dangerous, it certainly could be worth a try, although it should be kept in mind that stomach acid will destroy any protein allergen in honey. Remember that honey should not be given to children 12 months or less because of the rare but serious risk of infantile botulism.

www.uamshealth.com/?id=867&sid=1

CHAPTER VII
GERIATRIC ISSUES

A. ALZHEIMER'S DISEASE, THE SILENT EPIDEMIC

Everyone knows someone who suffers from Alzheimer's disease. At the present time, it is estimated that 5.3 million Americans have the disease, which is already the 6th leading cause of death in the United States. Patients may show only mild memory loss, which can then progress at variable rates to the complete debilitation of the end-stage disease. It is estimated that there are about 83,000 patients with Alzheimer's in Louisiana at this time, a number which will swell to over 100,000 by 2025. Around 1,400 people die from Alzheimer's in Louisiana alone each year, a figure that underestimates the real number of cases.

The impact of the disease for the patient, their entourage and the society is staggering. Patients may be functional in the beginning, but as the disease progresses, patients become less able to satisfy their own needs. The average annual per person medical costs for someone with Alzheimer's disease are around $33,000, over three times greater than for those without the disease ($10,000). It is estimated that the total dollar costs of Alzheimer's amount to $148 billion dollars a year, a figure that will grow as the number of cases increases with our aging population.

Besides the personal and economic impact of the disease, its effect on family members is often overwhelming. Caregivers of Alzheimer's patients are largely unpaid. Their responsibilities increase with time and become a full time 24 hour-a-day commitment, often with minimal assistance. In Louisiana, it is estimated that there are 160,000 Alzheimer's caregivers, who annually devote around 140 million hours of unpaid care worth around 1.5 million dollars annually. Because of the huge responsibility, physical, emotional and economic, associated with the care of Alzheimer's patients, it is not rare for the primary caregiver to sicken or even die before the person for whom they are caring, a huge and avoidable tragedy.

As individuals and a society, we must recognize the increasing burden of Alzheimer's disease. We must recognize the health concerns not only of the patient, but also of the caregivers and extended families. Denial of the effects of the disease on both the patient and family is not helpful in decision-making. Home health and hospice services need to be used when appropriate and necessary. Local chapters of the Alzheimer's Association provide an excellent resource. They can be located by consulting with the state (www.alz.org/louisiana) and national organizations (1-800-272-3900 and www.alz.org).

Although there is no cure for Alzheimer's disease at this time, the ultimate goal is to eliminate it through research, while still providing and enhancing care for the sufferers and their caregivers. The ticking time bomb of Alzheimer's disease will not go away, but perhaps can be defused by a collective social effort.

www.cdc.gov/aging/aginginfo/alzheimers.htm

http://www.alz.org/

B. LONG-TERM CARE:
THE IMPENDING TSUNAMI

America is aging rapidly. The famous "baby boomers" will turn 65 between 2011 and 2029, with about 10,000 turning 65 every day. Senior citizens will increase in numbers from 35 million in 2000 to 71 million in 2030. In the next 20 years, there will be an increase in 70% of those 85 and over.

Of these senior citizens, many will have multiple health issues (68% or more will have a lifelong probability of becoming disabled), and among those, many will require long-term services and supports (LTSS). For better or worse, most (87%) of those needing LTSS will receive them from unpaid family members. The typical profile of such an uncompensated caregiver is female (58%), 50 or older (66%), employed (47%) and caring for a parent (38%) for three years or more (44%).

For those without a devoted family member, there is always the option of paid long-term care in a nursing home or assisted living. The number of those requiring such services is currently over 13 million and will more than double to 27 million by 2050. Of those who reach 65, 70% can eventually expect to need long-term care services and at least 40% will enter a nursing home at some time.

Stays in such facilities can be expensive and prices vary from around $60,000/year in Louisiana to $162,000/year in Manhattan. Nursing homes care for some very sick individuals and, although severity of illness varies, 25% of all deaths in the U.S. occur in nursing homes. Deaths in nursing homes are expected to rise to 40% by 2020. In fact, of those patients who die in the nursing home, the average length of stay is only five months, testimony to severity of illness and social attitudes about death at home rather than about quality of care.

Since long-term services and supports are expensive, whether in a nursing home or community-based, most low income seniors run out of money. In fact, 34% of seniors already live at or below 200% of the poverty level and cannot hope to cover nursing home or assisted living costs. Of the $357 billion dollars spent each year on long-term services and supports, Medicaid is the primary payer (40%), while Medicare post-acute care covers 21%, and the rest is covered by other public or private sources (25%) or out-of-pocket (15%).

Even though Medicaid spending has been shifting toward community-based care (less than 20% in 1995 to over 40% in 2011), states vary widely in their home and community based spending (HCBS). Louisiana spends only 27% on HCBS, higher than the 16% in Mississippi but far lower than the 75% spent in Oregon.

The economic impact of long-term care in Louisiana is also significant. Long term care facilities employ 41,820 direct employees and provide $1.1 billion in labor income, with direct economic impact of over $2.2 billion. The demand for such facilities, regardless of the increase in home and community based services, will swell with the aging population.

Since most "Baby boomers" can expect to need long-term care in their lives, they also need to plan ahead for those paid services. Long-term care insurance is available, although almost 80% of those who purchase it have over $100,000 in available cash or stocks. If you intend to purchase such insurance, the price increases significantly with age, from about $1,900/year for someone 55 or younger to around $3,500/year for those aged 70 to 74. Interestingly, around 9% of those who purchase long-term care insurance let their policies lapse within a year of purchase.

Whether from a personal or national perspective, it is best to anticipate the needs of age and plan for the necessary expenses. The great dilemma in the United States is that we already spend 17% of our gross domestic product on medical care and increased expenditures risk breaking the national bank. That being said, we have an obligation to insure that the elderly can spend their golden years in some degree of comfort and with adequate medical oversight. How we achieve that goal defines our values as a nation.

American Health Care Association/ National Center for Assisted Living (Economic Impact of Long Term Care Facilities) www. ahcancal.org/research_data/trends_statistics

Kaiser Foundation (A short look at long-term care) http://kff.org

http://kff.org/infographic/visualizing-health-policy-a-short-look-at-long-term-care-for-seniors/

http://news.morningstar.com/articlenet/article.aspx?id=564139

C. DEPRESSION AND THE ELDERLY

Contrary to popular belief, depression is not a normal part of aging. While the multiple changes in later life (i.e. physical disabilities, loss of independence, retirement, death of loved ones and friends) may contribute to depression, it is never "normal to be depressed." In addition, depression, while it is sometimes more difficult to diagnosis in the elderly, is treatable and yields satisfactory results. Much of the secret of successful treatment lies in making the diagnosis and then getting the appropriate medications for an adequate length of time.

Of 35 million people in the United States who are over 65, about 6.5 million of them suffer from depression. Over 10% of Louisianans over 65 self-reported being depressed at least once in their life and 7% reported frequent mental distress. Depression in the elderly often masquerades as other illnesses (or may co-exist with them), including Alzheimer's disease, cancer, thyroid disease, some forms of arthritis, cardiac problems or many others. The symptoms of depression can include a host of non-specific conditions such as memory loss, inability to concentrate, insomnia, confusion, social withdrawal, irritability and many non-specific physical complaints.

Although depression does not have characteristic laboratory or radiological tests, it is important to rule out the numerous physical causes of depression with appropriate lab tests and x-ray results, usually including an MRI of the brain. Once important physical causes are ruled out, treatment options can include a variety of anti-depressant medications in at least four or five different categories. Since all medications can have significant side effects, doses must be titrated to the elderly to avoid preventable reactions and potentially life-threatening drug-drug interactions.

Any medication treatment regimen should be started low and increased gradually, with an expected improvement rate of over 80%. When a satisfactory response is achieved, it is imperative to keep on the medication for six months or more for a first depressive episode and often up to two years or more for recurrent episodes. Many people will stop medication because they "feel better," only to slip back into depression within weeks of stopping. Because anti-depressants affect the body's chemistry (altering neurotransmitters), it takes time for them to work and stopping them abruptly can precipitate unwanted physical and mental side effects. Drug regimens can be enhanced by psychotherapy by trained personnel and occasional require electro-shock treatments in particularly dangerous and refractory cases.

Depression in older Americans can be life threatening, with 14.3/100,000 of those 65 and older dying by suicide (16% of all suicides), the rate being highest among non-Hispanic white men. Sadly, many depressed elderly will seek help prior to committing suicide: 20% having seen a doctor the day they kill themselves, 40% the same week and 70% the same month. Depression may also be associated with and enhanced by substance abuse, either with alcohol (a known depressant) or any number of chronic narcotic pain relievers, prescribed or otherwise.

If you know someone who seems depressed, please have him or her evaluated by an appropriate professional. If they are suicidal, it is a medical emergency and 911 should be called. Make sure other medical conditions have been eliminated and make sure that treatments for depression are age-appropriate and monitored. The causes for depression in the elderly are multiple, but so are the successful treatments, which always include enhanced social networking and supports. Remember, depression is never a normal part of growing old!

http://www.cdc.gov/aging/mentalhealth/depression.htm

http://www.cdc.gov/prc/prevention-strategies/program-helps-elderly.htm

D. FALLS IN THE ELDERLY: CONSEQUENCES AND PREVENTION

As people age, their risk of falling increases, as does their risk for serious fall-related injuries. Decreased muscle tone, problems with vision, arthritic changes and medication or alcohol-related side effects all conspire to make the golden years more treacherous. For those 65 and older, one third will fall each year (60% of those at home) and most will not even mention it to their physicians. Falls are nonetheless the leading cause of injury-related deaths in this older age group. There were over 2 million fall-related injuries treated in the emergency room in 2010 and over 600,000 of those patients were hospitalized.

Of those thousands of elderly fall victims, about 2% will suffer a hip fraction. This comes to over 300,000 hip fractures a year (or 25,000 per month). Of those, 70% are in women, most of whom have some degree of osteoporosis (thinning of the bones). Of all hip fracture victims, 25% will die within a year of some combination of medical complications directly or indirectly related to their fracture and subsequent treatment. Although women are more likely to suffer hip fractures, older men are about a third more likely to die secondary to a fall. Whites are twice as likely to die from a fall as African-Americans. The total death count from unintentional falls in the elderly is over 20,000 a year, many of those related to traumatic brain injury resulting in cerebral contusions or subdural hematomas, clots on the brain.

In short, falls can be fatal and with the increase in the elderly population, prevention is the best medicine. Decreasing and strictly supervising medications and alcohol intake is imperative. Many drugs cause side effects and drug-drug interactions become more complex with increasing age and the number of medications. Since most falls occur at home, that environment must be made "elderly safe." That means removing loose rugs, clutter, wires, cords and dangling curtains. Adequate lighting is especially important, especially in halls and stairways. Grab bars and handrails should be installed and non-skid mats placed in bathrooms and kitchens. Shoes should be rubber-soled.

Fear of falling only decreases activity, resulting in reduced muscle tone and impaired balance, both of which increase instability. Regular exercise is imperative if at all possible. Inactivity also aggravates osteoporosis, a contributing factor to hip fractures, especially in women. A bone density test will determine if the bones are excessively thin and many treatment options exist. That being said, the indiscriminate use of calcium and vitamin D supplements has been implicated in an increase in cardiovascular disease in some studies. Use of calcium supplements in men is now being discouraged unless they have proven osteoporosis (something which is much less common in males.) While women do not seem to have an increase in heart disease related to calcium use, it seems wise to limit calcium supplementation to vitamin D alone, or calcium in that group of women with documented osteoporosis.

http://www.cdc.gov/HomeandRecreationalSafety/Falls/adultfalls.html

E. ELDER ABUSE: A NATIONAL EPIDEMIC

Abuse of the elderly has reached epidemic proportions in the United States and is likely to worsen in the future with the aging population. Bureau of Justice Statistics reveal that around 6 million cases were reported in 2010, and that represents only the tip of the iceberg. Over 80% of cases are not reported at all. About 9.5% of all persons over 60 will suffer some form of abuse, mostly by their own adult children or spouses (68% of cases). In fact, their own descendants killed 42% of all murder victims over 60.

So what is elder abuse? Abuse takes many forms and can be physical, emotional, sexual, and financial or may take the form of neglect or abandonment. It can come from those caring for the elderly person, or be categorized as self-neglect, often complicated by ignorance or dementia. Because of their diminished physical and mental capacity, the elderly are particularly susceptible to all forms of abuse. In addition, worsening intellectual capacity, including dementia, may make the older person prone to paranoia, angry outbursts and debilitating social isolation, which only aggravate the risk of abuse.

Caregivers themselves, burdened with increased responsibilities, may also be impaired by lack of education, poor coping skills, depression, lack of support and even substance abuse. The volatile combination of a difficult elder and an impaired caregiver makes abuse a likely outcome.

Since this is a common problem, family members, friends and neighbors, as well as all health professionals, should be attentive to this possibility. Bruises, broken bones, unexplained genital trauma or sexually transmitted diseases, regressive behaviors (rocking, withdrawal, or avoidance), can all be clues of physical, sexual or psychological abuse. Sudden, unexplained drops in bank accounts or extensive credit card charges can indicate financial abuse. Property, cash or identities may be stolen and wills, titles, and other legal documents altered.

Other suggestive behavioral signs with respect to caregivers can include humiliation, criticism, blaming or threatening their elderly charges.

Caregivers may limit contacts with the outside world, notably with friends, neighbors and home health personnel, and can intentionally or unintentionally limit services including, food, medications, and personal hygiene. Observers should always be on the lookout for elderly who appear undernourished, dirty, inappropriately dressed or wearing the same clothing repeatedly, washed or not. Unscrupulous health care professionals can also overcharge, underserve, or overprescribe to the elderly for financial gain.

Elder abuse is not rare, but is often difficult to identify. In addition, the abused person may be unwilling or unable to report such abuse for fear of retaliation or abandonment. Because elder abuse is a common problem, reporting is simple and all 50 states have laws protecting the elderly. The Elderly Protective Hotline in Louisiana is 1-800-259-4990 and for out-of-state problems, it is 1-225-342-9722. Since 14,000 cases occur each year in nursing homes and other long-term care facilities, such incidents need to be reported to the Long Term Care Ombudsman in Louisiana at 1-866-632-0922 or 1-225-342-7100 for out of state reports. We all have a responsibility to stop this disgraceful national epidemic.

http://www.cdc.gov/violenceprevention/elderabuse/index.html

F. SUBSTANCE ABUSE AND THE ELDERLY

Substance abuse has become distressingly common among the elderly, who are already becoming a larger segment of our society. There are currently 35 million people over 65 years of age in the United States and that number will increase significantly with the arrival of the long-anticipated Baby Boomers. Substance abuse affects around 17% of people 60 and older and that number is likely to double by 2020.

Sadly, the acceptance of substance abuse, whether it is with alcohol, benzodiazepines or pain relievers, has increased with time and now has achieved epidemic proportions. Aging Baby Boomers come with a different attitude toward substance use and abuse, colored by their experiences in the 60's and 70's. There has also been a simultaneous explosion in the use of all prescription medications, including pain (opiates) and anxiety (benzodiazepines) relievers.

Why are the elderly so subject to substance abuse? First, they have more medical conditions that require treatments. While older Americans represent only 14% of the population, they consume 25% of all medications, some of which lack appropriate medical indications. Second, they are often suffering from depression associated with retirement, loss of loved ones, physical and mental disabilities and isolation. Self-medication with easily obtainable substances, such as alcohol and over-the-counter sleep preparations, represents an irresistible temptation. Third, their substance abuse is either not recognized by family and medical providers, or it is tolerated as being one of an elderly person's remaining pleasures. Physicians diagnose around 60% of younger substances abusers in their clientele, but only 37% of elderly abusers. Fourth, biological changes in the elderly make them more susceptible to the effects of alcohol and other drugs due to changes in their metabolism and body mass.

Why should this be important? First, the direct cost of treatment for addictive problems in the elderly is staggering and already exceeded $250 million in the early 1990's. Second, alcohol and benzodiazepine use increase the risk for slips and falls, as well car accidents in those elderly who still drive. Third, alcohol alone is a depressant and causes a host of medical issues including nerve damage, liver damage and an increased risk for early dementia. Older male alcoholics have among the highest rates of suicide of any population group. Fourth, elderly abusers often go into withdrawals in the hospital and prolong lengths of stay and increase hospital costs significantly.

What can be done? First, recognition by family and medical personnel is essential. Second, treatment is possible and should be encouraged. Letting Granny or Grandpa enjoy their drinks (or even their marijuana) puts them at significant risk. Don't be an enabler. Third, treatment programs do exist and the elderly respond as well or better than younger substance abusers.

Take Granny's shopping bag of medications to the doctor for review and removal of unnecessary or dangerous products. Don't ignore danger signs of social isolation, depression, and instability and memory loss. Let's identify this high-risk group and get them the help they deserve to make their lives longer, richer and more fulfilling.

Taylor, M.H. and Grossberg, G.T., "The Growing Problem of Illicit Substance Abuse in the Elderly: A Review." Prim Care Companion CNS Disord. 2012; 14(4): PCC.11r01320. Published online 2012 July 12. doi: 10.4088/PCC.11r01320 PMCID: PMC3505129 www.ncbi. nlm.nih.gov/pmc/articles/PMC3505129

Matthews, R. "As Elderly Population Surges, So Will Substance Abuse." ACEP News Elsevier Global Medical News, May 2010. http:// www.acep.org/content.aspx?id=48626

G. SMOKING AND THE ELDERLY

Older Americans have among the highest smoking rates of any age group in the United States. Over 50% of men smoked in the mid-1960s and half again as many had previously smoked. Although the number of current smokers in all age groups has declined to fewer than 20%, at least 9% of Americans over 65 still smoke. Many have adopted a lackadaisical attitude that "the harm is already done," and "it won't do any good to stop now." While the first statement may be true, the latter is surely false.

Why is smoking so destructive? First, smoking destroys elastic tissue in the lungs, blood vessels and skin, resulting in COPD (Chronic Obstructive Pulmonary Disease), atherosclerosis (hardening of the arteries) and even wrinkles. Atherosclerosis causes increased rates of heart attacks, strokes, peripheral artery disease and delayed wound healing. Smoking-related hardening of arteries in the brain accelerates and aggravates cognitive dysfunction (memory loss), including Alzheimer's disease, which occurs a third more often in long-term smokers. It also increases cataract formation, contributing to decreased vision and impaired driving.

Second, the cancer-causing effects of smoking produce most lung cancers and increase the numbers of other cancers as well (mouth, throat, esophagus, bladder, cervix and pancreas). Third, smoking interferes with bone formation and predisposes to osteoporosis (weak bones), which increases the risk of fractures following a fall. Falls, fractures and complications related to surgery and hospitalizations can be life-ending experiences for the elderly.

Smoking kills 438,000 people in the U.S. each year, or 20% of all deaths. Half of all smokers will die from their habit. Since the evil effects of smoking increase with age, 70% of these smoking related deaths occur in people over 60 years of age. COPD, 90% of which is smoking related, is the fourth leading cause of death in the United States and equals the deaths from cardiovascular disease. A smoker has a 60% greater chance of dying from a heart attack than non-smokers and male smokers will die from a stroke twice as often as their non-smoking peers. Life expectancy is reduced around 14 years in smokers, cancelling out the hopes of a long, happy and healthy retirement.

Although older smokers are less likely to try to quit, those that do will succeed more often. When older smokers quit, those with COPD breathe more easily and those with circulatory problems will have less pain and can ambulate better. Quitters will add anywhere from 1.4 to 3.4 years of life expectancy. Following a tobacco cessation program, which often includes both counseling and medications, can increase success rates in the elderly (now at less than 5%) just as it does in younger smokers. The QUIT LINE offers free, individualized help at 1-800-QUIT-NOW (1-800-784-8669). A simple phone call may add quality years to your life. It's never too late to stop smoking.

http://www2c.cdc.gov/podcasts/player.asp?f=6787

H. HINI (SWINE FLU) AND THE ELDERLY

There was a great deal of interest about novel H1N1 and its effects on the elderly during the pandemic of 2009-2010. Much of this interest was generated by the fact that those over 65 years of age were not included in the initial priority groups for vaccination. That decision was based on the fact that 84% of the confirmed H1N1 cases were in those less than 24 years old and that initial supplies of the vaccine were limited.

By mid-2010, the CDC estimated that there had already been around 47 million cases of H1N1 in the U.S. population. Of those, around 16 million (34%) were in those 0-17 years old, 27 million (57%) were in those 18-64, and only 4 million (8.5%) were in those 65 and older.

The CDC also estimated that, by the same date in mid-2010, there were around 213,000 hospitalizations related to H1N1, of which 71,000 (33%) were in those 0-17 years old, 121,000 (57%) were in those 18-64, and only 21,000 (10%) were in those 65 years and older.

As far as deaths were concerned, CDC estimated there were 9,820 H1N1 related deaths in the U.S. during the pandemic period (mid-2009 to mid-2010). Around 1,090 (11%) occurred in those 0-17 years old, 7,450 (76%) in those 18-64, and only 1,280 (13%) in those 65 and older. In other words, although someone 65 and above was less likely to get H1N1 than their younger counterpart, they were more likely to die from the disease if they contracted it (five times more likely than someone in the 0-17 year age group) because of their underlying fragility.

It was speculated that those born before 1950 benefited from some residual immunity from previous H1N1 exposures. Those 65 years of age and older, however, suffer from other medical conditions that make them susceptible to influenza complications. As vaccine became more available, the age restrictions for those able to get the H1N1 vaccination were lifted. There was considerable interest in getting the H1N1 vaccine among the elderly, who are already more sensitized to the benefits of influenza vaccination in general, based on their past medical experience and information.

Although fears of a more serious pandemic, with a much higher case fatality ratio, did not materialize, there were still around 10,000 deaths in the U.S. from attributed to H1N1. There were also some fears about the vaccine itself, which, while almost understandable with a "new" vaccine, were not justifiable. The vaccine preparation was not new, although the organism was "novel." In addition, very careful follow-up of the millions of H1N1 doses given worldwide failed to show any significant side effects. Three separate monitoring systems, the Vaccine Adverse Event Reporting System (VAERS), Vaccine Safety Datalink (VSD) and the Active Surveillance for Guillain-Barré Syndrome and others were all used in the United States and confirmed H1N1 vaccine safety.

Everyone, both in and out of the medical field, was thankful that H1N1 did not prove more deadly. We should not, however, decrease our vigilance. Flu viruses have built-in mechanisms for mutation and are constantly undergoing changes. Potential for a mutated H1N1 with much higher mortality is certainly possible. Annual flu vaccination is still always recommended. H1N1 displaced other flu viruses for the subsequent flu season, but it is only a matter of time before some more virulent strain develops, possibly related to the ever-present Avian Flu in Southeast Asia. An influenza pandemic of the same catastrophic intensity of the 1918 Spanish Flu is a statistical inevitability, however no one knows when it might occur or where it might originate.

Public interest in novel H1N1 waned given the mild clinical manifestations and low case-fatality ratio, but it would be tragic to lose any patients to what is a vaccine-preventable illness. During the H1N1 Pandemic, we were far from the 35,000, mostly elderly patients, who die each year due to seasonal flu (less than half that number died during the H1N1 Pandemic). That is a tragic figure we hope to avoid every year by aggressive vaccination of all elements of the population older than 6 months. Medical decisions should always be based on risk-benefit analyses and here the benefits of vaccination (saving lives) far outweigh any negligible risks associated with the vaccine.

www.webmed.com/cold-and-flu/features/swine-flu-and-the-elderly

I. HIV/AIDS AND THE ELDERLY

When one thinks of HIV/AIDS, the elderly are not the first group that comes to mind. It is estimated by 2015, however, that over 50% of those living with HIV/AIDS will be 50 or older. Those over 50 also represent over 10% of newly diagnosed cases of HIV/AIDS or around 75,000 cases/year. Three percent (3%) of all newly diagnosed HIV/AIDS cases are over 60 years old.

Complicating the situation is a chronic racial disparity among older HIV/AIDS cases, with around 50% of them being in African-American and Hispanic individuals of both sexes. In fact, in the over 50 group, African-Americans have 12 times and Hispanics 5 times the rates of HIV/AIDS as whites. Among women over 50, the number of cases increased by over 40% in five years, $2/3^{rd}$ infected by their partner and $1/3^{rd}$ by injectable drug use.

What has led to this explosion of cases among the elderly? In fact, there are two reasons for this increase. The first is related to HAART (Highly Active Anti-Retroviral Treatments), which have prolonged the lives of those infected at an earlier age. HIV/AIDS, while not curable, has become a highly treatable disorder. These multi-drug therapies, complicated and expensive as they are, have increased the life expectancy of HIV/AIDS suffers by decades.

The second explanation is related to the increase in new HIV/AIDS cases in the elderly. Because of treatments for erectile dysfunction (ED), heavily advertised to the general public in direct-to-consumer marketing, it has become more common for the elderly to engage in sexual activity. Because women over 50 are usually menopausal, worries about pregnancy vanish and unprotected sex becomes more common. Since women live longer than men and the rate of divorce has steadily increased, many women find themselves as widows or divorcees with new partners whose sexual history is unclear or unknown.

To aggravate the situation, early symptoms of HIV/AIDS may include vague fevers, weight loss, fatigue, arthritic pains, rashes or respiratory problems that may be more common in the elderly and explained away by other incorrect diagnoses. This is particularly true of AIDS related dementia, which may mimic Alzheimer's disease and not be considered until other medical conditions develop.

Unlike younger sexually active adults, older individuals have not been educated about AIDS or encouraged to undergo regular testing. According to Bill Rydwels, a senior citizen and AIDS activist in the Chicago area, "People over 50 come from a generation where the discussion of sex was an under-the-table thing. Nobody wants to discuss the sexual habits of older people. It's the concept that older people stop having sex, and it's just not the reality."

Older adults, especially those who are sexually active, should always consider the diagnosis of HIV/AIDS. You need to verify the status of your partner(s), and use condoms (male or female) during intercourse. If you have received a transfusion between 1978 and 1985, a delayed diagnosis of HIV is always possible. As we tell younger adults, ignorance is not bliss and silence is not golden. Get tested and consider the possibility of HIV/AIDS even if you are a senior, sexually active or not.

Testing is provided with no out-of-pocket expense at CLASS or any Office of Public Health location throughout the region or state.

http://www.nia.nih.gov/health/publication/hiv-aids-and-older-people

J. ANTIBIOTIC USE IN NURSING HOMES

There are over 15,000 nursing homes in the United States, 282 of which are located in Louisiana. Nationally, there are 1.6 million nursing home residents, with 30,000 in Louisiana alone. Most (6 out of 7) residents are 65 years of age or older and many suffer from one or more chronic medical conditions. When so many elderly individuals with so many medical problems are grouped together, the chances of someone receiving antibiotics increase greatly. In fact, over 70% of nursing home residents receive an antibiotic every year, costing anywhere from $38 to $137 million annually.

With such a concentration of germs and antibiotics, the risk of developing or being exposed to antibiotic resistant organisms skyrockets. Many residents will be "colonized" with bacteria, meaning they carry the germ on their skin, nasal secretions, sputum or urine without showing any signs of infections. Around 250,000 nursing home residents nationally have some infection, and 27,000 have an antibiotic resistant organism. To aggravate things, many frail nursing home residents can have recurrent hospitalizations and may return to the nursing home with multiple resistant organisms including Methicillin Resistant *Staphylococcus aureus* (MRSA), vancomycin-resistant enterococci (VRE), and various resistant Gram-negative bacteria. Many have in-dwelling devices such as feeding tubes and Foley catheters that increase risks of long-term colonization. Sometimes these patients are treated with prolonged courses of antibiotics, indicated or not, thus aggravating resistance issues.

Of the antibiotics given in the nursing home setting, 32% goes for urinary tract infections, 33% for respiratory infections, 12% for skin infections, and 10% for other sites and 13% undisclosed. From one third to one half of elderly residents will have a positive urine culture without showing any signs of infection. A reported "positive" culture may be treated inappropriately, increasing the chances for bacterial resistance and/or development of *Clostridium difficile*. This latter organism, while not resistant itself and frequent with all antibiotic use, can cause terrible recurrent diarrhea and is very difficult to eradicate from the environment.

How can providers, administrators, residents and their families reduce this growing danger of antibiotic resistance? First, cultures should be obtained before starting antibiotics and the treatment modified depending on the results. Second, treatment should also depend on the patient's symptoms, not just the culture results. Third, length of treatment should be as short as possible and should not be initiated at all if the disease is likely to be viral (i.e. cold, flu, viral gastroenteritis.)

Louisiana falls in the top of the charts for per capita antibiotic use in the United States, while the U.S. exceeds European averages. It is far easier and quicker for a doctor to prescribe antibiotics than to explain to anxious patients and their families why it might not be necessary, or even harmful, to do so. Doctors are also subject to fears of litigation for "delays in treatment" and "denial of chance by withholding treatment." Despite justifiable physician anxiety, the CDC still recommends an "antibiotic timeout" when culture results become available, especially in the absence of corresponding symptoms. There should always be careful reflection about the risk/benefit ratio to the patient and the general public prior to any antibiotic prescription. We should all "Get Smart about Antibiotics" while we still have them around for use. Injudicious use of antibiotics, especially in long-term care treatment facilities, may lead to a time when none are available to fight life-threatening infections.

http://www.cdc.gov/getsmart/healthcare

K. DECADE OF DANGER: 55 TO 64

The waning years of professional life should be spent enjoying the fruits of a life's labor in anticipation of a well-deserved retirement. For many Americans, however, the critical years between 55 and 64 become a perilous bridge from private insurance to the enhanced security of Medicare. Most Americans between the ages of 55-64 (86%) still benefit from some form of health insurance. The majority are employer-based insurance (63%), followed by a much smaller group with individual health insurance (6%), and some with early Medicare or Medicaid (16%). That still leaves 14% of Americans between 55 and 64 without any form of insurance.

Although the Affordable Care Act should extend some form of insurance to this group of uninsured, the critical decade from 55-65 years of age is still fraught with dangers. Around 41% of the uninsured between 55-64 years old report unmet medical needs or delayed care in 2010, an increase of 10% since 2003. During that same time period, those with insurance reported only 17% with unmet needs and delayed medical care in 2010, an increase of only 6% from 2003.

Those critical pre-Medicare years see a simultaneous increase in medical problems, associated with a decrease in earning potential related to changes in the job market. Such an unfavorable alignment of the stars can be fatal. Not only do a third of uninsured people have problems paying medical bill, but almost 40% find themselves $5,000 or more in debt with respect to those bills.

Since a disproportionate percentage of those pre-elderly without health insurance are low income, a higher percentage of those are African-American. The constellation of no coverage and limited means helps explain in part the increased mortality among African Americans in this age group. Those lucky enough to qualify for Medicaid can look forward to significant reductions of their problems paying for prescription drugs (only 8%) or paying medical bills (only 6%), down from over 40% in those without insurance.

When seniors eventually qualify for Medicare, there is still a serious problem if they cannot afford a Medicare supplement. Around 14% of those with Medicare, but no supplement, still have problems affording medications, and 18% have a problem paying medical bills. With a Medicare supplement, this drops to only 5% having medication cost issues and only 6% with problems paying medical bills.

Central Louisiana has a higher than national average of uninsured (20% vs. 14%), and a correspondingly larger number of uninsured in the 55-64 year old group as well. Up to now, everyone dreads the thought of losing his or her job (and health insurance) prior to the magic Medicare age. While seniors may wave their newly minted Medicare card with a combination of triumph and palpable relief, it's not long before the realities of the necessity of Medicare supplemental insurance sets in.

While the Affordable Care Act may offer some relief, it will certainly not decrease the cost of medical care, estimated at $8,000 per capita for all ages and double that for those over 75 years of age and older. The combination of increased age and infirmity, coupled with the increasing cost of medical treatments in general, may prove fatal to the nation's economy. Attempting to eat and drink in moderation, while maintaining an active lifestyle and a healthy weight is still the best prescription of all. Prevention is always the best medicine!

"Cost and Access Challenges: A Comparison of Experience between Uninsured and Privately Insured Adults Aged 55-64 with Seniors on Medicare." Kaiser Family Foundation, Medicare Policy, May 2012. http://kff.org/health-costs/report/cost-and-access-challenges-comparison-of-experiences/

L. THE AFFORDABLE CARE
ACT AND THE ELDERLY

Since most individual over 65 already benefit from Medicare, the implementation of the Affordable Care Act may seem rather abstract. One of the more direct impacts for the elderly appears to be the closure of the infamous "donut hole," the point at which Medicare recipients previously lost medication coverage and had to pay full price until a new threshold was achieved.

What is less obvious is the ultimate impact of the financial considerations of expanded insurance benefits to those previously uninsured segments of the population. This group represents 14% of the American population or around 47 million people. The number is disproportionately higher in Louisiana, where 20% of the adult population is uninsured (around 400,000 or more).

Most medical providers will readily admit that having some form of medical insurance for everyone is a good thing. In fact, the vast majority of providers recognize the problems associated with the uninsured, which tend to use the nation's emergency rooms as their primary source of medical care. Because hospitals cannot legally turn away any emergency case (EMTALA), hospitals become the unwilling providers of last resort to those who may have significant neglected medical conditions.

The hope now is that the previously uninsured will be affiliated with a stable pool of primary care providers that will keep patients healthier and out of the emergency rooms, a notoriously expensive venue for treatments of any kind. While the theory is admirable, the reality may prove less so. Those with Medicare can usually locate a primary care provider. Those with Medicaid, who represent 25% of the population in Louisiana, have a much greater challenge. There has been the state system of hospitals and health units that serve any constituents, but these were expensive systems, subject to periodic budget cuts, and now totally transformed into "public-private partnerships." Many individual private providers do not take the uninsured or Medicaid due to reimbursement issues. Given the choice of patients, the most economically desirable from a provider's perspective are the privately insured, then Medicare, and lastly, Medicaid. Some uninsured actually pay office visits in cash rather than incur the cost of insurance.

Access, therefore, has been and will remain an issue for Medicaid patients even though there are incentives to increase reimbursement to primary care physicians and those groups and individuals who chose to or must accept Medicaid. The access issue will be aggravated in Louisiana when another 400,000 or more individuals swell the 1.2 million who already receive Medicaid (increasing this group to over 40% of the state population). The same phenomenon will take place nationwide, although to a lesser extent in more prosperous states with lower numbers of indigent citizens.

The other issue remains the cost of increasing coverage nationally. Theoretically, implementation of the Affordable Care Act will save the country a trillion dollars in ten years. This pales in comparison to the 2.7 trillion dollars spent annually on health care in the United States. Our per capita medical expenditures of over $8,000/year is more than double that spent in other developed countries that already achieve near universal coverage. We already spend over 17% of our gross national product on health care and this may increase to 20% or more in the next few years even before complete implementation of the Affordable Care Act. Most other developed countries spend 10% or less, setting the stage for worsening of our international competitive position and aggravation of the national debt, both legitimate economic concerns.

When it becomes obvious that costs will escalate despite our best-laid plans, existing programs, such as Medicare, may well lose their privileged positions. The healthcare pie may have to shrink and Medicare, Medicaid and other federal healthcare programs may have to shrink with it. Will this happen? No one knows for sure. But the complexity of the problems of health care, combined with the unsustainable costs of our current medical delivery system, do not bode well for the future.

http://www.aarp.org/content/dam/aarp/health/healthcare reform/2013-07/aca-factsheet-for-65-aarp.pdf

http://www.hhs.gov/healthcare/prevention/seniors/

M. ALEXANDRIA, LOUISIANA:
CITY FOR SUCCESSFUL AGING?

In 2012, the Milken Institute evaluated large and small metropolitan areas around the United States to determine their geriatric friendliness. This involves an analysis of a number of indicators in categories including General, Financial, Transportation, Community Engagement, Employment, Living Arrangements, Health-care and Wellness. Each of these, in turn, contains a number of distinct parameters.

So how does Alexandria, Louisiana rank? Out of the 259 "Small Metro" areas, Alexandria ranked a very favorable 28/259 (36/259 for those between 65-79 and 11/259 for those over 80.) Such a remarkable performance merits some closer scrutiny. One thing that distinguishes the results is the disparities of the scores depending on the indicator. While Alexandria ranks 12/259 for "Financial," the city only ranks 227/259 for "Community Engagement." Even within an indicator, the spread was remarkable. For "Financial," we rank 11/259 for the number of banks, but fall to 231/259 for the percent of those over 65 who are below poverty. A similar disparity exists within "Community Engagement," where we rank 11/259 for the number of libraries per capita, but only 252/259 for the rate of senior volunteerism.

A similar discrepancy exists between "Healthcare" and "Wellness." For the former, which reflects the availability of health resources (doctors, hospitals, hospice, rehabs, nurses, etc.), Alexandria ranks 19/259. For "Wellness," the ranking falls to a much less impressive 203/259, a category that includes diabetes rates, Medicaid eligibility rates, % of seniors living with family members, Alzheimer's cases, life expectance and some other values. That paradox between the high "Health-care" and low "Wellness" reflects the poor health of the population in general. Louisiana regularly ranks 49/50 among states in the America's Health Rankings.

So is Alexandria a good place to grow old? Our city, like much of the South, represents a dichotomy. Even within a single category, there is often a wide disparity of results, from very high to very low. This reflects some of the complexities of a city with lots of bank, hospitals, and nursing homes, but also with a lot of crime, poverty, diabetes and those who have not completed high school or college.

Taken as a whole, Alexandria still ranks fairly high among small metro areas and is still a good place for aging. There is still, however, plenty of room for improvement in the reduction of disparities that tend to aggravate and perpetuate some of the less favorable statistics. In addition to "objective" rankings, those human assets that citizens bring to the city also help determine the quality of a city. One can be miserable and unhappy in Sioux Falls, South Dakota (#1 among small cities), as much as in Alexandria, Louisiana. And there will be very contented people in the small town ranked 259th (Morristown, Tennessee) in the Milken Institute scale. Perhaps we all just need to work a little bit harder to close the gap between our strengths and weaknesses.

Participating in the civic life of the community enhances both individual and public health outcomes. Since Alexandria ranked a dismal 252/259 for senior volunteer rates, there is a great opportunity for improvement. Seniors can help make this a better town in which to live and enhance their own quality of life in the process. Every town, including Alexandria, can be the best town to live in.

http://successfulaging.milkeninstitute.org

www.americashealthrankings.org

N. TESTS, PROCEDURES AND TREATMENTS THAT SENIOR CITIZENS DO NOT NEED

Senior citizens represent a growing segment of the population. With age comes a multitude of medical issues often involving complicated tests and treatments. In this era of high technology, the growing complexity of such tests might seem a boon to health. More, however, is not always best. Physicians and patients must always weigh the costs and potential harms due to a test against the benefits of the particular procedure. There is a point at which the dangers of testing (or the dangers of procedures resulting from that testing) exceed the potential benefits. To make the situation more complicated, the real interest to society is a test's value, which is the quality, divided by the cost. Since some tests or procedures may give some benefit, but the cost of that benefit is excessive, it is literally not worth doing.

In order to help consumers navigate this minefield of choices, the American Board of Internal Medicine (ABIM) has requested its component organizations to list some tests, procedures and treatments that should NOT be done. These are not arbitrary recommendations, but based on research and consensus opinions of the organizations that determine standards of care. Here are some of those results more applicable to senior citizens.

The American Geriatrics Society (AGS) does NOT recommend feeding tubes in patients with advanced dementia, but prefers oral assisted feedings. They do NOT recommend antipsychotic medications or benzodiazepines as first choices for behavior issues in demented patients. They do NOT recommend trying to achieve a glycosylated hemoglobin (Hg A1C) of less than 7.5% for diabetic control in those 65 or older. (In other words, looser diabetic control is not detrimental as life expectancy decreases.) The AGS does NOT recommend use of antibiotics to treat asymptomatic bacteriuria (germs in the urine) in older men and women under most circumstances.

The American Gastroenterological Association does not recommend repeat colonoscopies sooner than 10 years when a first, high-quality test is negative (no polyps) and for five years if there are one or two small (less than 1 centimeter) polyps. They recommend the lowest effective dose of acid suppression medication (proton pump inhibitors or H-2 receptor antagonists) for reflux. And they do NOT recommend repeat CT scans of the abdomen for "functional abdominal pain syndrome" (when no structural lesions are identified.)

The American Urological Association (AUA) does NOT recommend the use of testosterone in men with ED (erectile dysfunction) and normal testosterone levels. They do NOT recommend treating patients with elevated PSA values with antibiotics in hopes of lowering the PSA. Bone scans are NOT recommended in patients with "low risk" prostate cancer (PSA < 20 and Gleason score 6 or less).

The Society of Cardiovascular Computed Tomography (SCCT) does NOT recommend coronary artery calcium scoring in patients with known coronary artery disease, including stents and by-pass grafts or as a screening tool in asymptomatic adults with no family history. They also do NOT recommend coronary CT angiography for screening in asymptomatic adults.

The American College of Obstetricians and Gynecologist do NOT recommend Pap tests in those over 65 years of age. And they do NOT recommend screening with CA-125 or pelvic ultrasound for ovarian cancer in asymptomatic women with no family history.

In short, although this list is long and complex, it only represents some of the many tests that are NOT recommended. It is imperative that the patient becomes actively involved in the process of diagnosis and treatment. With every test or procedure, you can and should ask, "Is it necessary and what will you do with the results." You do not want to suffer the consequences of a test that was not indicated in the first place. The cost to you and society may be just too high.

http://www.choosingwisely.org/doctor-patient-lists/

O. END-OF-LIFE DECISIONS: MEDICAL, LEGAL AND FINANCIAL

The end of life is a critical period for anyone. While no one wants to get there, death comes to all of us and our loved ones just as surely as taxes. Discussions surrounding impending death are painful and difficult at any time. The person may or may not realize that they are about to die and the family may or may not be willing to bring the subject up. To make matters worse, the timing of life's end is never an absolute certainty and with few exceptions, no one knows the day and hour of their demise. Some people, who are expected to die in the very near future, will rally and live days, weeks or months more.

In addition, all those complex social and psychological (not to mention financial) issues that have often not been addressed in the past suddenly rush to the forefront and demand immediate attention. This is a volatile and potentially explosive period. Guilt, anger, resentment, greed and selfishness can co-exist with love, devotion, appreciation and a genuine desire to be of service. Relatives from near and far may converge on the bedside and long-simmering resentments can bubble up in the exhaustion and confusion of the end-of-life scenario, especially when it is a prolonged process.

None of us wants to face our death or anyone else's, but we should all want to make this important life transition as smooth as possible. The patient and family may not want to, but confronting some of the multiple complex decisions prior to death can save an enormous amount of grief for everyone. What are some of these decisions?

One of the first should be that of having a standard will. Watching families agonize (or fight) over what their loved one "would have wanted" is a painful experience. A standard last will and testament can avoid much of that uncertainty and conflict. A frank discussion of who wants what may seem cold and heartless, but it is even worse having siblings bitterly fighting over a silver tea set or a piece of furniture. A trust may also be indicated in some circumstances, although it is a more complex document requiring special legal input. It also requires the naming of a trustee, a position of relative power and authority, which itself may pose a problem for the siblings.

Everyone should also create a living will, a document that clearly delineates the level of care they want to receive as they approach death. Do they want any resuscitative procedures? CPR? Tube feeding? A breathing machine? Antibiotics? What should be done medically and how far the doctors should go, and under what circumstances, should all be clearly addressed. The drama of a distant relative, who insists on prolonged futile care while the rest of the family wants their loved one "just made comfortable," is a formula for disaster. Deciding to place a feeding tube and then deciding not to use it or remove it is as traumatic as placing a person on a ventilator and then having to remove it at some point. If these decisions have been made in advance, the burden is taken off family members who are no longer guessing at what the patient may or may not have really wanted.

There are also decisions about who will have Power of Attorney when and if the patient becomes physically or mentally unable to make their own decisions. This also extends to the Medical Power of Attorney, a person designated to make only medical (and not financial) decisions. Everyone may think they will remain lucid until the point of death, but that is the exception and not the rule. It is estimated that 5.4 million Americans suffer from Alzheimer's disease now and that figure will only increase with the aging population. Such individuals cannot make reasoned decisions despite the best information. Voluntarily designating someone with Power of Attorney also avoids the difficult problem of establishing competency, a complicated legal (not medical) designation.

Doctors are often the witnesses to horrendous scenes of family conflict, played out at the bedside of a dying family member, just as they are witnesses to heart-warming scenes of solidarity and love. Addressing wills, living wills, Power of Attorney, Medical Power of Attorney, and even the decision of when and how to initiate hospice measures can all be made in advance. Such forethought brings peace and closure to loved ones who can concentrate on grieving and not be left making burdensome, sometimes conflict-generating end-of-life decisions.

Koppel, A and Sullivan, S. "Legal Considerations in End-of-Life Decision making in Louisiana." Ochsner J. 2011 Winter; 11(4): 330-333. PMCID: PMC3241065

www.ncbi.nlm.nih.gov/pmc/articles/PMC3241065/

CHAPTER VIII
INFANTS, CHILDREN
AND ADOLESCENTS

A. MY KID DID WHAT? HIGH RISK BEHAVIOR AND ADOLESCENTS

Every parent dreads the call from a neighbor, friend, school official or police officer telling them their child has committed some outrageous, high-risk act. Whether it is substance abuse, driving while distracted or drunk, truancy, or pregnancy, all such behaviors seem incomprehensible to the adult mind. Yet they occur every day by the thousands. In the best of circumstances such behavior may result in a reprimand or a simple medical intervention, in the worst of cases, they may result in death.

Why then does this high-risk behavior occur in adolescents? Why does the United States have one of the highest teen pregnancy rates in the developed world (39/1,000 live births) with over a million girls getting pregnant each year? Why do 23% of high school students report binge drinking within the last 2 weeks? Why do 35/100,000 young people die each year from unintentional (70% motor vehicle accidents) and intentional injuries (around 44% MVAs and 20% homicides).

It is estimated that over 60% of teens engage in some sort of dangerous behavior every year. Many of these activities have been the target of aggressive educational prevention campaigns, both in schools and in the general media. Has there been any improvement? The answer is yes, but not enough. There has been a decline in births to teens over the last decade in all races. There has also been a reduction in teens that drink and drive. Yet the problems still persist despite significant educational attempts. Why?

The answer to this perplexing dilemma lies in the nature of the teenage brain. At the same time that young people are becoming physically mature, enough to engage in sexual activity and drive, there is a lag in the development of their frontal lobe (the anterior portion of the brain). That part of the brain is responsible for judgment and impulse control. It allows young people to refrain from risky behavior, with immediate gratification, in deference to delayed gratification because of perceived long-term benefits. An example might be a decision to refrain from getting pregnant because child rearing could interfere with completion of an education necessary for a better, more highly paid and responsible job.

The frontal lobe develops fully from late adolescence into the early twenties, a time when most parents will agree that adolescent behavior mysteriously improves. In fact, there is no mystery, just neurobiology. There may have been some evolutionary primate advantage to having young apes take the risks of establishing new colonies. But that advantage has long since disappeared. Unreasoned risk taking offers little advantage and creates lots of real problems.

What then is the solution to this neuro-biological discrepancy? It is impossible and undesirable to lock adolescents up from 13 to 25 years of age, a time when much important learning and socialization takes place. What can be done is threefold. First, educate adolescents both at school and at home in the consequences of high-risk behaviors. Second, engage in role-playing exercises that ingrain better decision making into young people. And third, try, as much as possible, to reduce exposure to circumstances where adolescents can get into trouble, something which requires parental discretion and supervision. Without all three components, success will be limited. With all three components, there is no guarantee, but a better chance of risk reduction. So rather than saying "My kid did what?" after the fact, give adolescents real facts beforehand, role play high-risk scenarios, and keep your kids out of obviously risk prone environments.

http://www.acpeds.org/the-college-speaks/position-statements/parenting-issues/the-teenage-brain-under-construction

B. BREASTFEEDING AND LOUISIANA: ROOM FOR IMPROVEMENT

Whether you are a parent, grandparent, or just a casual observer, nothing evokes the tenderness of motherhood more than breastfeeding. Although not all women succeed in breastfeeding, the benefits for newborns are astonishing. Breastfeeding reduces infections, reduces the risk of sudden infant death, and even reduces the risks of infant and child obesity. It also reduces maternal risks of breast and ovarian cancers.

Despite all of these documented advantages, only around 56% of Louisiana women initiate breastfeeding. Only 20% continue at six months and barely 10% make it to a year. This is opposed to U.S. statistics of 75% initiation, 43% at 6 months and 22% at one year. The statistics for African-American women in Louisiana are disproportionately worse. Only 30% of African-American women initiate breastfeeding, while only 13% continue at 6 months and less than 5% continue until a year.

This racial disparity in breastfeeding is not unique to Louisiana. Nationally, only 60% of African-Americans initiate breastfeed, but only 28% continue at 6 months and around 13% continue to a year. The reasons for this racial disparity are not clear, but it is worse in Louisiana than in the United States in general. That African-Americans in Louisiana breast-feed at only about half the rates of African-Americans nationally may have many social and historical roots, but it is a clear call to action for those in policy-making and public health circles.

Breastfeeding, despite its obvious advantages, faces obstacles of social acceptance, workplace accommodations, and inadequate support in the family and at all levels of medical intervention. While Louisiana has only a handful of "Baby-Friendly" hospital facilities as of 2013 (as opposed to Nebraska with over 20%) (www.babyfriendlyusa.org), it does have the GIFT program, which certifies hospitals that implement successful practices related to infant feeding and maternal-infant bonding. There are currently 21 "GIFT Certified" birthing facilities in

Louisiana, with more applying every year. Several medical facilities are also close to attaining "Baby-Friendly" status.

To increase the number of mothers who breast-feed, hospitals should have a written breastfeeding policy, with administrative buy-in and training for all personnel. Mothers should be informed about and assisted in breastfeeding, initiated within an hour of birth. Mothers and infants should remain together if at all possible and the infant should feed on demand. Supplemental feeding and pacifiers should be avoided and formula-containing gift bags for new mothers should be eliminated. Support groups for lactating mothers should be encouraged. A perennial, but not insurmountable, stumbling block appears to be the use of "free" donated formula from manufacturers, which must be refused by "Baby-Friendly" institutions. Once overcome, however, the coveted "Baby-Friendly" status can be attained and is well worth the efforts.

Breastfeeding should also be introduced with pre-natal care and continued through the hospital experience and into the pediatricians' offices or Office of Public Health (or other WIC providers). Persistent, coordinated education and support, specifically targeted at the African-American community, should help improve breastfeeding statistics in Louisiana. Improvements in infant and maternal health will inevitably follow.

Older adults play a critical role in encouraging their own children or grandchildren to initiate breastfeeding. Once started, a supportive entourage, especially older women in the family, help increase the length of time that breast-feeding is continued. In either case, the infants, their mothers and the society as a whole are all beneficiaries.

www.cdc.gov/breastfeeding/

C. SUDDEN INFANT DEATH SYNDROME (SIDS): AN OFTEN PREVENTABLE TRAGEDY

Sudden Infant Death Syndrome (SIDS) refers to the unexpected death of a child less than one year of age. The loss of a child is a terrible tragedy from which parents almost never completely recover. It is out of the natural order of things for children to die before their parents, a fact which intensifies both the length and severity of grieving when an infant dies.

SIDS is not a rare phenomenon, with 80 babies a year dying in Louisiana alone. Central Louisiana had the sad distinction of being ranked number one in SIDS (1.9/1,000 live births) out of all of the Louisiana public health regions in 2012. Although it is impossible to completely eliminate the possibility of a sudden infant death for unexplained reasons, there are some clear risk factors that can be reduced or eliminated.

First, babies should be placed on their backs (not on their stomachs) to sleep, on a firm mattress, without pillows, cushions, toys or bumper pads. This may seem like a sad and unfriendly sleeping environment for the infant, but it is the best and safest one and has been shown to reduce the risk of SIDS. The infant should be dressed in light clothing in a comfortable (not over-heated) room.

Second, co-sleeping, a cultural tradition in some families, increases the risk of infant death through unintentional smothering. Some well-intentioned mothers will engage in breast-feeding (a very positive action) in the bed while lying down (a poor position). An exhausted mother can easily fall asleep in such a position, unintentionally smothering their infant. Such avoidable rollover deaths are sometimes erroneously classified as SIDS deaths.

Third, premature and low birth weight babies are more susceptible to SIDS. Every effort should be made to reduce prematurity through appropriate spacing of children, avoiding teenage pregnancy, and eliminating smoking. Elective deliveries prior to 39 weeks should be eliminated. Young smoking mothers with multiple children are at a particular risk for prematurity and the sudden infant death that might result.

Smoking is also an independent risk factor for SIDS, whether it is the mother or others in the household. Smoking cessation will help not only the adults, but the infant and other children in the household. Louisiana offers a number of programs including the tobacco cessation Quitline (1-800-QUIT-NOW) and www.QuitwithUsLa.org. Other states offer similar programs.

Back-to-sleep, no co-sleeping, a firm, empty crib, no smoking, avoiding teenage pregnancy and eliminating elective deliveries prior to 39 weeks are all mainstays of reducing SIDS. Perhaps there will always be the rare infant who dies an unexplained death, but we can all do what we can to avoid those risk factors that have been shown to increase it. Even one avoidable infant death is too many.

www.sids.org/

http://www.cdc.gov/SIDS/index.htm

D. GUNS AND KIDS:
A LETHAL COMBINATION

Guns, when mixed with children and adolescents, make for a deadly combination. In a country where there are as many guns as people (310 million firearms), the pairing of kids and guns becomes increasingly common. Although not every household contains a gun (62% do not), over 3.3 million children live in homes where a gun is kept, sometimes loaded and unlocked. Over 75% of first and second graders from gun-owning households know where a gun is located in their home and most are physically capable of pulling the trigger.

The presence of a gun in the home, especially if it is unlocked (31.5%) and loaded (21.7%), drastically increases the incidence of accidental injury (4 times), suicide (3-5 times) or homicide (3 times). In fact, for every time a gun is used in the home for self-defense, there are 11 suicide attempts, seven assaults and homicides and four unintentional shootings (mostly by friends and siblings). The toll of death and injury astonishes, with over 2,600 deaths by firearm and over 15, 500 non-fatal injuries among children and teens in 2010 alone.

While motor vehicle accidents (MVAs) still kill more young people each year than other causes, there are disturbing racial disparities with firearms. The devastation from guns, not MVAs, was the leading cause death among African-American males between 15 and 34 in 2009. In 2010, almost half of the deaths and injuries from firearms were among African-American children and teens even though African-Americans represent only 15% of the youth population. Between 1963 and 2010, firearms killed over 52,000 African-American youths (36% of the total deaths in this age group.) African-American children and teens are 8.5 times more likely than Whites to be injured by guns and 17 times more likely to die from gun-related homicide. African-American youths, aged 15-19, are 30 times more likely to die from gun-related homicide than Whites in the same age group.

All of this tragedy comes with a huge price tag, above and beyond the grief to family and friends. In 2000 alone, the cost from gun-related deaths and injuries to children, teens and adults amounted to $17.4

billion (around $1 billion in direct medical costs and $16.6 billion in lost productivity.) The Children's Defense Fund claimed that these costs had risen to $174 billion by 2010 (a tenfold increase), with 8.4 billion in direct medical costs and $53.5 billion in lost productivity. Hospitalization costs from nonfatal firearm assaults were estimated to be around $23,000/case and self-inflicted injuries were over $7,000. These hospital costs must be multiplied by the 15,575 children and teens seen in hospital ERs for gun-related injuries in 2010 (40% of whom required hospitalization.)

When compared with other developed countries, the United States distinguishes itself by having a firearm suicide rate for children between 5 and 14 years of age that is 8 times higher and accidental firearm injuries 10 times greater than countries with comparable incomes. For young people between 15 and 24, the U.S. firearm suicide rate is a remarkable 35 times greater than other developed countries.

The American Academy of Pediatrics (in their 2012 policy statement) recommended the following steps to reduce this needless slaughter: (1) Advocate for the strongest legislative and regulatory approaches for prevention of firearm injuries and deaths. (2) Educate parents about the need for safe storage or removal of firearms from the home (". . . the safest home for a child or adolescent is one without firearms."). (3) Encourage trigger locks, lock boxes, gun safes, and safe storage legislation. (4) Restore the ban on assault weapons. (5) Support the research on firearm-related injury prevention, including the NVDRS (National Violent Death Reporting System).

Parents, healthcare professionals and policy makers all need to work together to address the preventable problem of gun-related injuries and deaths among children and teens.

http://pediatrics.aappublications.org/content/130/5/e1416.full

http://www.chop.edu/healthinfo/firearms-injury-statistics-and-incidence-rates.html

http://www.childrensdefense.org/programs-campaigns/protect-children-not-guns

E. ATV USE: RECREATIONAL DANGERS

ATV riding is a popular form of recreation in the United States, with over 8 million of them in use. Louisiana, as "Sportsman's Paradise," has a significant number of such vehicles. Although they are popular, they are not a risk-free form of recreation, especially for children. The Region VI (Central Louisiana) Child Death Review Panel of the Office of Public Health has the sad responsibility of reviewing deaths among children from 1 to 14 years of age and ATV accidents continue to be a major source of morbidity and mortality in CENLA and around the United States.

Nationwide, there were 2,620 ATV-related deaths from 2003 to 2006 (44 of them in Louisiana) or about 800 a year. Five hundred and ninety one deaths (or 22 percent) of them were in children younger than 16. From 2007 to 2010, there were an additional 385 deaths in children under 16 in the U.S. Louisiana ranked 19th/50 states for the absolute number of deaths associated with ATVs from 1982-2009 (228) although we are only 25th in population.

Besides the horror of death, from 2000 to 2010, there were over 1 million ER visits related to ATV injuries, over 25 percent of those in children younger than 16 and around 10 percent in children under the age of 12. Over half of the significant injuries were fractures of the upper or lower limbs or skull, with another 30% involving intracranial or crush injuries. Around 800 devastating spinal cord injuries occurred in children under 16 from 2000-2004 in the U.S.

The total cost of ATV-related hospitalizations amounted to over 1.25 billion from 2000-2005. Over the same time period, the cost associated with ATV deaths rose from 673 to 973 million dollars for adults and from 1.98 to 2.39 million in children. Spinal cord injuries occurring from 2000-2004 cost 24 million in medical expenses. The cost of all ATV-related deaths and injuries is estimated at $3,500 per ATV sold in the U.S. and those sales exceed 1 million vehicles a year.

One death is an unbearable tragedy for the families involved. When the death is a child, the pain and sorrow are almost unimaginable.

To avoid such tragedies, all parents need to follow some elementary rules: It is illegal to ride an ATV on a public road or paved surface (RS 32:299). Children under 6 should never ride an ATV. No child under 16 should operate an adult sized ATV (engines larger than 90 cc). Helmets should always be worn, as well as gloves, boots, goggles, long pants and long-sleeved shirts (despite our hot and humid climate). Passengers should not be allowed. Children and adults should complete approved ATV safety courses. Parents should always supervise children operating ATVs. Similar rules apply to off-road vehicles as well.

Remember, ATVs can and do roll over, especially in rough terrain. They are not designed for passengers and can weigh up to 800 pounds. Although ATVs and off-road vehicles may be an integral part of the rural way of life, parents, the manufacturers, law enforcement, educators, and public health representatives must work together to reduce the terrible and avoidable injuries and loss of life associated with their use, especially among children. www.atvsafetynet.org

U.S. Consumer Product Safety Commission (www.cpsc.gov) (search "ATV")

F. DRIVING TO DISTRACTION: DANGEROUS AT ANY AGE

Whether you are a 16 year old with their first drivers license, or a seasoned 60 year old with hundreds of thousands of miles of driving, you can be a victim of injury or death as a result of distractions while driving. Distractions come in three forms: visual (looking away from the road), manual (doing other things with your hands) and cognitive (thinking about other things.)

Distractions were involved in 20% of accidents in 2009. In those accidents, 5,400 people died and 448,000 were injured. Cell phone use was directly related to over 1,000 of these deaths (about 18% of the total) and 24,000 of the distraction related injuries. Not surprisingly, with the proliferation of hand-held electronic devices, the percentage of fatalities associated with distraction has risen from 7 percent in 2005 to around 11 percent in 2009.

Use of a cell phone "regularly" or "fairly often" while driving is reported in 40% of those aged 18 to 29. Regular cell phone use while driving drops to only 8% in those 60 years and older. In the same 18 to 29 year old group, over 25% report texting or e-mailing while driving (as opposed to only 3% of 60 year olds and older), a practice which places them at extreme risk.

Despite the dangers of texting or e-mailing while driving, over 1% of young drivers (16 to 24 years old) have been directly observed to be manipulating hand-held electronic devices at the wheel. This seems to be higher in the South than in the West and Midwest. Using such devices while driving appears to be slightly more common in females than males.

At any given time, someone is using a hand-held cell phone in 672,000 vehicles, which greatly increases their chances of a fatal accident. This person is more likely to be young, female and live in the South. That being said, driving distracted at any age and in any location can prove a fatal choice.

Response to this epidemic of electronic distraction varies from state to state and from country to country. While there is no nationwide federal ban against cell phone use while driving, the practice is banned and subject to ticketing without another offense in at least 10 states and the District of Columbia. In Louisiana, the use of cell phones while driving is banned for school bus drivers and also for novice drivers (as a secondary offense). Many European countries ban the use of cell phones while driving as a matter of public safety, with fines of hundreds of Euros.

Whatever the legal statutes, distracted driving is deadly driving. Use of a cell phone, whether hand-held or hands-free, reduces a driver's reaction time as much as a blood alcohol level of 0.8 percent. Some people, who would not dream of drinking and driving, will use a cell phone without a second thought.

Don't put your life or the lives of other drivers at risk. Don't call and drive. Don't text and drive. And don't drink and drive either. No phone conversation or text message is worth your life. Put down the phone and keep your hands on the wheel.

www.fcc.gov/guides/texting-while-driving

www.textinganddrivingsafety.com/texting-and-driving-stats/

G. OF CHICKS, DUCKS AND LITTLE TURTLES

When Easter rolls around, there is an almost overwhelming temptation to buy one of those fuzzy little chicks or ducklings for your children or grandchildren. The rising popularity of backyard poultry has only increased the temptation, since many people now have their own backyard flock. While little chicks are tempting, the same holds true for that cute little turtle that comes from the street vendor or that you might even catch in your own back-yard stream or bayou. Before you succumb to temptation, however, remember that chicks, ducks and little turtles share one thing in common, the bacterial infection, *Salmonella*. In fact, birds, reptiles and amphibians (frogs and toads) are susceptible to *Salmonella* infections and may not show any signs of illness while they are still carriers.

Children (younger than 5) are more susceptible to *Salmonella* infections than adults and can become seriously ill. In older individuals, the disease usually causes fever, nausea, vomiting, abdominal cramping and diarrhea within a few hours of exposure (often 12 or less). The symptoms last from four days to a week and usually resolve without treatment, although antibiotics are sometimes required for more serious or prolonged cases.

Salmonella, whether in children or adults, is one of the most common intestinal infections, causing thousands of cases each year, many of which go unreported even though it is a reportable disease. Diagnosis depends on identification of the bacteria in the stool, although it may also be found in the urine and blood in some individuals. Since 1990, there have been 45 Salmonella outbreaks related to live poultry, with 1,563 illnesses, 221 hospitalizations and 5 deaths. There were eight outbreaks nationwide in 2012 alone and one in Louisiana in 2013 with 14 cases.

Cute little chicks, ducklings (or turtles) are simply not worth the risk. If you or your children handle live poultry, reptiles or amphibians, please wash your hands thoroughly with soap and water. Do not let children under five handle live birds or reptiles, since they are prone to put the animal or their contaminated hands in their own mouth.

If you have a pet bird or reptile, do not let it roam around the house, especially in areas where food is handled.

There is surely nothing more miserable than spending the week after Easter in the emergency room or hospital with a case of massive, painful diarrhea. While it is illegal to purchase turtles smaller than four inches in diameter, chicks and ducklings are readily available in feed stores and elsewhere. Every year there are multiple cases of infected children from their avian or reptilian pets. You do not want your child or grandchild to be one of them.

Hanzlik, K. "Multi-State Salmonella Outbreak Associated with Baby Chicks Includes Louisiana." LA Morbidity Report, Jul-Aug, 2013, Vol. 24, No. 4

www.cdc.gov/salmonella/

H. AUTISM AND THE CHILDHOOD VACCINATION CONTROVERSY

Autism is a general term for one of several manifestations of "autism spectrum disorders." Parents dread the possibility that one or several of their children might develop this problem. The mystery involving the origins of this disorder only adds to the challenges and frustrations of raising a child with this disease. Parents and researchers alike are driven by a desire to know what causes autism and how it could be prevented or cured. Although a combination of genetic and environmental causes have been proposed, there is still much uncertainty, and much corresponding research, surrounding the topic. To add to the distress and sense of urgency is the reality or impression of the increasing number of cases of autism. Whether this increase in numbers is due to increased public and medical awareness or a real increase in cases is also still unclear.

The association between autism and vaccinations sprang into the public consciousness in 1998 with the publication of an article by Dr. Wakefield and his colleagues in the prestigious British scientific journal, *The Lancet*. Dr. Wakefield claimed that vaccination with MMR (Mumps, Measles and Rubella vaccine) caused autism, as well as a specific form of enterocolitis (an intestinal disorder later dubbed "autistic enterocolitis.") What followed was an explosion of worldwide publicity, referred to later by critics as "science by press conference."

Alarmed parents all over the world, and specifically in the United Kingdom, began refusing to vaccinate their children. Confidence in MMR and other childhood vaccines plummeted and the resulting controversy swept around the planet (via the internet.) It generated more than 1,200 articles in 2002 alone, exceeding publications about all other scientific studies. A flurry of research resulted in at least 14 major publications that eventually discounted any link between childhood vaccinations, specifically MMR, and autism.

That did not stop the proliferation of lawsuits and parental distrust that still continues to this day. Various ill-informed or misleading physicians even proposed so-called "User-Friendly Vaccinations

Schedules" or "Alternative Vaccination Schedules," both of which expose children to unnecessary risks of infectious diseases. In the end, Britain's General Medical Council found that Dr. Wakefield acted "dishonestly and irresponsibly," "with callous disregard" for the children in the study and he was sanctioned and stuck off the medical register (losing his license to practice medicine.) His study, tainted by conflict of interest, was considered "the most damaging medical hoax of the last 100 years."

A similar controversy swirled around the use of the preservative thimerosal, added in multi-use vials of some vaccines. It contains ethyl mercury, which inhibits the growth of bacteria and fungus, contaminants that can cause serious or fatal infections. Mercury can be toxic, but the form that is incriminated is methyl mercury (not ethyl mercury), a substance that can be ingested in the flesh of certain fish and accumulates in tissues. Vaccines in the U.S., with the exception of some multi-dose vial influenza vaccine, no longer contain thimerosal. Even so, the cumulative exposure dose if all childhood vaccines contained thimerosal would be less than 3 mcg of mercury, an infinitesimal amount.

Fortunately, autism, while still mysterious in its origin, is not related to childhood vaccinations. The fact that autism develops at the same time that most childhood vaccinations are given has led to an unfortunate and inaccurate "guilt by association." It is hoped that the tremendous interest in autism, and support of research concerning its true causes and effective treatments, will result in a better understanding of this mysterious disorder.

Downs, M. "Autism-Vaccine Link: Evidence Doesn't Dispel Doubts," WebMD.

http://www.webmd.com/brain/autism/searching-for-answers/vaccines-autism

http://www.healthychildren.org/English/safety-prevention/immunizations/pages/MMR-Vaccine-and-Autism-What-Parents-Need-to-Know.aspx

CHAPTER IX
HEALTHCARE
OUTCOMES AND POLICY

A. LOUISIANA HEALTH RANKINGS 2013: 48ᵀᴴ WITH ROOM FOR IMPROVEMENT

United Health Foundation recently published its 2013 America's Health Rankings. All of the states are ranked according to a collection of "health determinants" (or factors) and "health outcomes." Determinants include many aspects of behavior, community characteristics, policy and clinical care that determine health outcomes (for example, diabetes, infant mortality, cardiovascular deaths, cancer deaths and premature deaths.)

Louisiana, with its high percentage of Medicaid (25%) and uninsured (20%) and its low median income ($40,000 vs. $50,000 nationally) has always struggled with its ranking. Since 1990, when the rankings first began, Louisiana has been 49ᵗʰ and 50ᵗʰ much of the time. Mississippi has helped boost Louisiana's ranking for several years, although sometimes we have been tied with our Southern neighbor.

We are in the fourth quartile (from 37/50 to 50/50) for the following health determinants (factors): low high school graduation rates, smoking, obesity, sedentary lifestyle, children in poverty, violent crimes, occupational fatalities, infectious diseases (including sexually transmitted diseases and HIV/AIDS), lack of health insurance, preventable hospitalizations, and low birth weight babies.

As far as health outcomes (related to morbidity and mortality) are concerned, we are in the fourth quartile (worst) for cancer deaths, cardiovascular deaths, premature deaths, diabetes, and poor self-reported mental health days.

On a more positive note, we are in the top half (best) for low binge drinking, high immunizations rates for children and adolescents, good numbers for primary care physicians and high per capita spending on public health (although it has dropped slightly). The latter distinction bears comment since it clearly indicates, much as does our high per capita expenditures on Medicaid, that the money spent does not necessarily translate into better health determinants or outcomes. Poor outcomes can be related to social and economic disparities more than absolute spending. The obvious exception appears to be childhood vaccinations, where Louisiana is a remarkable 25/50 in our immunization rates for children and 6/50 for adolescents, largely due to a progressive and comprehensive electronic record for vaccinations (LINKS) and a well-organized immunization program.

Although Louisiana has made modest progress in high school graduation rates (now 68.8%), we still remain significantly below the national average (around 80%). Ambitious efforts are also underway to transform the Medicaid delivery system with the implementation of Bayou Health, private administrators of the significant funds devoted to Medicaid. It is hoped that these new private partners will succeed in making health care utilization more cost effective and achieve better results. Mental health services are also being reformed to come under the auspices of local governing entities, Central Louisiana Human Services District in our region, and an outside mental health administrator, Magellan. The Birth Outcomes Initiative targeted prematurity by reducing unnecessary deliveries prior to the critical 39-week date and appears to be improving outcomes.

In short, Louisiana still ranks poorly, but positive initiatives have been undertaken to improve our dismal statistics. Sometimes it takes years, if not decades, to see the statistical fruits of such initiatives. It is hard to ask for patience, however, given the long history of poor outcomes and the massive amounts of money and manpower that have been devoted to improving them.

Perhaps the most ominous development has been the inexorable increase in obesity in the state (now 50/50) that threatens to submerge the healthcare delivery system in a tidal wave of poor health, especially uncontrolled diabetes. As with all health problems, all we can do is to study the facts, apply evidence-based improvement techniques where possible, and not be discouraged by our significant opportunities for improvement.

www.americashealthrankings.org

B. PARISH HEALTH RANKINGS 2013: CENLA'S PROBLEMATIC PROFILE

Each spring, the Robert Wood Johnson Foundation, in collaboration with the University of Wisconsin Population Health Institute, releases the County (Parish) Health Rankings & Roadmaps. These statistics are intended to stimulate local health and state health departments to focus on problem areas within their states.

These statistics are separated into "Health Outcomes," based on mortality and morbidity results (often a year or more late) and "Health Factors," based on a conglomerate of health behaviors (30%), clinical care (20%), social and economic factors (40%) and physical environment (10%). Each of the health factors is based on a number of components, too numerous to mention here but readily available on www.countyhealthrankings.org.

Over the years, Central Louisiana's eight parishes have been divided into four groups relative to one another and the other 64 Louisiana parishes. As far as "Health Outcomes" are concerned, LaSalle (8/64) and Vernon (14.64) rank in the top quartile, Winn (23/64) and Rapides (31/64) rank in the second quartile, Grant (38/64) and Avoyelles (44/64) fall in the third quartile, and Concordia (59/64) and Catahoula (61/64) rank in the bottom quartile of Louisiana Parishes.

Since "Health Outcomes" are largely determined by "Health Factors," there is a rough correlation between the two. That being said, none of our eight parishes fall in the top quartile of health factors, while Rapides (17/64), LaSalle (22/64) and Vernon (24/64) rank in the second quartile, Grant (35/64) and Winn (46/64) fall in the third quartile, and Avoyelles (51/64), Concordia (54/64) and Catahoula (60/64) fall in the lowest quartile.

Over the past four years (since the 2010 County Health Rankings), there has been little variation in these rankings. LaSalle and Vernon Parishes consistently top the list of parishes with the best health outcomes, while Catahoula and Concordia have proven the worst. Over the last four years, there have been no remarkable trends in health outcomes rankings except perhaps a decline from 2 to 14/64 for Vernon and an improvement from 35 to 29/64 for Winn Parish. When health factors are considered, LaSalle and Rapides top the list as the "healthiest" places to live, while Avoyelles, Catahoula and Concordia consistently appear to be the "unhealthiest." Since 90% of this determination is based on personal behaviors, access to care and socio-economic factors, it is easier to understand these rankings.

While West Feliciana was 1/64 in its health outcomes and St. Tammany (1/64) topped the list for health factors, these rankings must be taken in context of the Louisiana's health ranking of 48/50 states (America's Health Rankings 2013). Being first among the last (or next to last) may not be much cause for celebration. Having said this, Louisiana health remains a challenge, which can only be met by a concerted effort of public policy and individual commitment. Either alone will rarely achieve the desired goals of improvement in our parish (or state) health statistics.

www.countyhealthrankings.org

www.americashealthrankings.org

C. CENTRAL LOUISIANA: SOME BASIC FACTS

Central Louisiana (Office of Public Health Region VI) comprises eight parishes (Avoyelles, Catahoula, Concordia, Grant, LaSalle, Rapides, Vernon and Winn). The regional population is about 300,000, almost half (120,000) living in Rapides Parish. This part of Louisiana, like much of the state, distinguishes itself by the three adjectives: poor, unhealthy and under-educated. That being said, there are those who are wealthy, healthy and well educated, but they do not represent the majority. The disparities between the haves and have-nots may well contribute to these persistent poor health outcomes.

The per capita income of Central Louisiana is around $24,000, which translates into around 25% of the population living in poverty. This corresponds to the same percentage that benefit from Medicaid, while close to 20% do not have any health insurance at all. Regionally, only around 68.8% of children finish high school and only around 10% go on to obtain a college degree (as opposed to 24% nationally). The combination of poverty and lack of insurance (or under-insurance) almost guarantees poor health outcomes.

Louisiana ranks 48/50 states in its health outcomes in 2013. Not surprisingly, Louisiana ranks 40th or above compared to other states for smoking (24.8%), obesity (34.7%), violent crime (496/100,000), chlamydia infections (697/100,000), lack of health insurance (19.6%), preventable hospitalizations (87.5/1,000 Medicare enrollees), infant mortality (8.1/1,000 live births), cardiovascular deaths (318.5/100,000) and cancer deaths (219/100,000) Adding to the deluge of grim statistics is the nation's highest murder rates (11.8/100,000) and incarcerations rates in the United States (800/100,000), disproportionately affecting African-Americans. To complete the tableau, Louisiana ranked #1 for syphilis, #2 for gonorrhea, #4 chlamydia and #4 for HIV/AIDS rates in the United States in 2010. The figures vary only slightly since then, but Louisiana consistently remains in the top 5 states for STDs and HIV/AIDS.

Central Louisiana is not much different than the rest of the state, although our crime rates and STD rates are somewhat lower and our obesity rates are somewhat higher. Death rates in Central Louisiana exceed state averages for heart disease, stroke, and cancer. Over 60% of Central Louisiana's population is either overweight or obese. Over 30% of children fall into the same category, with black girls being the heaviest group. Overweight children have over an 80% chance of continuing on to become obese adults, who have higher rates of hypertension, diabetes mellitus, kidney failure and cancer.

Less than a third of Louisiana children aged 6-17 meet current federal physical activity levels and over 40% exceed recommended limits for screen time. Only 10% of Central Louisiana children eat three or more vegetables daily, but over 35% watch television three or more hours a day.

With our national health expenditures exceeding 2.8 trillion dollars a year (around 17% of the gross national product), and Louisiana being no exception to these increasing costs, solutions must be found to reverse the dreadful health outcomes that burden our nation, state and region. Every credible attempt to reduce obesity will pay dividends in decreased morbidity and mortality. Since the origins of our poor health outcomes are complex and multi-factorial, the solutions will likewise have the same diversity.

It is our hope that approaches that combine education, the arts, and physical activity provide the best opportunity to produce long-term results and reverse those trends that will result in children dying before their parents. It has been demonstrated that there is a direct correlation between enhanced social capital and improved health outcomes. Bringing together diverse populations in the context of a variety of non-traditional programs may help accomplish the goals of better health as a byproduct of enhanced social capital. Synergy between collaborative groups in efforts to enhance health also offers the best opportunity of success. Poverty, sickness and lack of education do not need to be the three adjectives describing CENLA, the heart of Louisiana.

www.americashealthrankings.org

www.countyhealthrankings.org

www.kidscount.org

www.louisianareportcard.org

http://www.rapidesfoundation.org/site/Portals/0/docs/2013%20 CHNA%20Report%20-%20Rapides%20Foundation%20Service%20 Area.pdf

D. THE ALPHABET SOUP OF CHANGE: ACA, CCN, ACO AND CSOC

In this era of dramatic changes in the medical landscape, the average citizen is bombarded with a series of acronyms, all essential to an understanding of our healthcare transformations.

The first one is **ACA** or the Affordable Care Act. It is a complex document, sometimes referred to as "Obamacare." It does many things, but one of the most important for Louisiana could be the huge increase in the number of patients with Medicaid. Although Louisiana has opted not to expand Medicaid at this time, it already has about 25% of the population under Medicaid. We also have around 20% who are uninsured. It is conservatively estimated that the full implementation of the ACA, including Medicaid expansion could result in an increase of over 400,000 new Medicaid patients in the state of Louisiana, or a total of around 40% of the total state population.

The United States, alone among developed countries, still has a significant percentage of uninsured (16% of the population) and decreasing the number of uninsured is universally recognized as a laudable goal. Yet two major problems arise: First, the cost of medical care in the United States already consumes 17% of the gross national product and consumes 2.8 trillion dollars a year. Second, many physicians have been unwilling to accept Medicaid patients, leaving them technically insured, but still without access to medical care.

That leads us to the second acronym, **CCN** or "Coordinated Care Networks," also know as Bayou Health plans in Louisiana. These are organizations that act as Medicaid intermediaries to which their affiliated providers submit their bills for services. There are two variants of these organizations. One variant of these Bayou Health plans operates as "shared savings" system in which the organizations benefit from hypothetical savings generated from improved health and reduced costs among their constituents. The second variant is that of Bayou Health plans that accept capitated payments (so much money per affiliated member per month). Their profit, if any, is derived from reduced expenses secondary to improved care. The more efficient the plan in generating savings, the more profit they can generate. The success of either variant of CCNs depends on the participation from providers, the inherent efficiencies of the network, and the amount the state is willing to devote to Medicaid payments in the first place. As of June 1, 2012, Bayou Health plans were implemented throughout the state, replacing previous single-payer Medicaid program.

That brings us to **ACO**s or Accountable Care Organizations. These are national models that combine insurers and providers, whether hospitals or physicians or others, in a system where the organization is accountable for certain quality results, achieved by a more coordinated and efficient allocation of resources and services. The better the results, the higher are the potential reimbursements to providers. Various financial incentives (and disincentives) are built into the system to encourage cooperation in the patient's best interest. Theoretically, the cost of care will decrease by improving prevention and decreasing wasteful duplications of services and avoidable hospital re-admissions.

That leads us to **CSOC** or "Coordinated Systems of Care." This is a Louisiana initiative to coordinate the care of high-risk youths among various providers, including the judicial system, Children and Family Services (formerly Social Services), the educational system and other community providers. Individual high-risk cases are managed in order to reduce the possibility of such clients falling between the cracks of various agencies. The system theoretically reduces the cost to society for those few cases that consume inordinate amounts of resources. In Louisiana, this **CSOC** has the name of "Eckerd's," a partner in the rollout of this concept in our state.

Confused yet? Yes, it is very confusing. The Affordable Care Act (**ACA**), Coordinated Care Networks (**CCN**) (i.e. Bayou Health), Accountable Care Organizations (**ACO**), and Coordinated Systems of Care (**CSOC**) are all parts of the complex new wave of health care initiatives. The hope is that they will finally help to bring some coherence into an inefficient and expensive system that has left us both bankrupt and unhealthy as a nation and a state. We may be forced to eat this alphabet soup (as opposed to chicken soup) to restore some health to our notoriously inefficient healthcare delivery system.

E. NOT ENOUGH PRIMARY CARE PROVIDERS?

Primary care providers, including family practitioners and general internists, form the backbone of the healthcare delivery system. They, along with nurse practitioners, physician assistants and other "mid-level providers" or "physician extenders," take care of routine and not-so-routine patient needs, usually in the outpatient setting. These are the caregivers with whom the patient forms a special bond and to whom they turn for advice or for referrals to specialty physicians.

It has been demonstrated that communities (or countries) with a higher proportion of primary care providers have less emergency room visits, less hospitalizations, higher levels of preventive care, including vaccinations and cancer screenings, and lower mortality rates. More primary care doctors equates to a healthier community, something that does not necessarily hold true for specialists.

Health, however, has not been the driving force in medical career choices. In the medical and other professions, economics and life-style considerations also drive decisions more often than altruism. Medical residents in internal medicine used to go into primary care about 50% of the time, but this number has dwindled now to less than 20%. Most internists now enter subspecialty training or become hospitalists (those who work exclusively in the hospital). Meanwhile, the number of family practice residents, who almost always stay in primary care (90%), has remained flat.

What drives this dwindling number of primary care providers? The answer is complex, but includes lower reimbursements, less professional prestige, mountains of complex rules, regulations and paperwork, demands of recertification, frenetic call schedules associated with sacrifices of family and personal time, and the horrors of litigation in our nightmarish medico-legal environment to name but a few explanations. Thus, incentives to remain in primary care have diminished, while incentives to leave it have increased.

Unfortunately, the aging population and the expansion of medical demand related to the Affordable Care Act mean that the need for primary care would only increase, just as the supply levels off or even declines. Reactions to this situation vary from dire predictions of doom and gloom to more nuanced interpretations. Some experts raise the alarm and recommend immediate changes in reimbursements and graduate medical education funding. Others feel those electronic medical records, medical homes, and an increased number of "physician extenders" will fill the void. In reality, however, most "physician extenders" work with sub-specialty doctors and not with primary care physicians.

No one, however, really knows for sure what the future holds, but what is known is that primary care providers play a positive, even crucial, role in the community's health. The ballooning of medical costs in the U.S. aggravates the turmoil in medical care in general. With 17% of our GDP consumed by our massive medico-industrial complex, spending more money is not a realistic option. More and more, the decision to reward or punish elements of our healthcare delivery system will depend of the cost effectiveness of that segment. Hospitals, recipients of the largest slice of healthcare pie, risk being "losers," while primary care providers may well come out as "winners." Primary care is cheaper, more efficient, gives enhanced bang-for-the-buck in preventive care and results in healthier communities. Despite that winning combination, the flight from a choice of a primary care career continues to accelerate. In fact, the loss of primary care physicians, such valuable resources to any community, occurs at a much higher rate than for subspecialists at any doctor's age.

What can reverse this trend? Shifting reimbursements, collaborations of multiple providers in medical homes, a more charitable approach to lifestyle and reductions in the constant dread of litigation will all help. The question remains as to whether we, as a society, are willing or able to make such difficult choices. If we can, however, we will all live in a healthier community. It is up to policy makers to align public interest with the clear advantages of adequate primary care.

Swartz, M.D., "The US Primary Care Workforce and Graduate Medical Education Policy," JAMA, Dec 5, 2012, Vol 308, No. 21, p 2252.

http://jama.jamanetwork.com/article.aspx?articleid=1475164&resultClick=1

"How Is a Shortage of Primary Care Physicians Affecting the Quality and Cost of Medical Care," American College of Physicians, A White Paper, 2008.

http://www.acponline.org/advocacy/current_policy_papers/assets/primary_shortage.pdf

Petterson, S.M. et al. « Projecting US Primary Care Physician Workforce Needs 2010-2025." Ann Fam Med. Nov/Dec 2012. Vol 10(6) p 503-509.

http://www.annfammed.org/content/10/6/503.abstract

F. UNINSURED AND THE AMERICAN MEDICAL SYSTEM, HOW MUCH CAN WE AFFORD?

Currently, we still have 47 million U.S. citizens, 14% of the population, without medical insurance, although this number may drop with the full implementation of the Affordable Care Act. The percent uninsured in Louisiana is closer to 20%, while another 25% of Louisianans have only Medicaid. Louisiana, like many other states, does not oblige physicians to accept any Medicaid patients, a situation which compounds problems of access to care for this insured, but underserved, segment of the population.

A former Department of Health and Hospitals Secretary spoke about the laudable increase in insured children in Louisiana, as well as alluding to the persistent problem of medical access. What was not mentioned then, but had spoken of on other occasions, is the problem of the spiraling cost of medical care in general. It is not a long-term solution to increase the number of insured under our current bank-busting system of medical delivery. The U.S. spends 2.8 trillion dollars a year on medical care, which represents 16% of the gross national product, over $8,000 per person per year. The amount spent on those 75 and older is over $17,000 per person per year. On the one hand, our per capita healthcare expenditures are around double those of other industrialized countries. On the other hand, our medical outcomes are not the best in the world, either in percent of insured citizens, longevity, cancer mortality, heart disease, infant mortality, sexually transmitted disease rates, or any other internationally recognized health parameters. The inescapable conclusion is that we do not have the best medical delivery system in the world, simply the most expensive.

With the expected future increases in medical spending in the U.S., we were on track to reach 20% of the gross national product by 2020 (or perhaps sooner), although there is some reassuring evidence that medical costs have begun to level off. This is still an unsustainable level of spending, even for the wealthiest country in the world. We have created a medico-industrial complex of many individuals who benefit from our healthcare delivery system, none of whom seem to be willing or able to see their portion of this great pie shrink. Yet shrink it must if the U.S. is to retain a competitive position in an increasingly global and competitive environment.

There is no one guilty party in the development of this strange and unacceptable situation. Deliverers of healthcare and health related services, as well as the general public, have all contributed to this sorry state of affairs. But as has been pointed out, simply increasing the number of insured individuals without changing the fundamentals of the system will only increase cost burdens without eliminating dysfunction. We must have the courage to engage in this critical debate at both a state and national level without forgetting that we are not operating in a vacuum, but in a global context. Each element of this 2.7 trillion dollar medico-industrial complex, as well as the general public, must decide whether they wish to remain part of the problem, or help by becoming part of the solution. Each person must decide whether they are willing to tolerate the backbreaking burden of healthcare expenditures on personal and a national level. If reductions must occur, then they should be done with a vision of equitable care and not simply to insure the health and prosperity of a few.

G. A MODEST MEDICAL PROPOSAL

In 1729, Jonathan Swift wrote "A Modest Proposal," his classic criticism of British indifference to the plight of millions of starving Irish. In it, Swift proposed that the Irish and their British overlords eat Ireland's starving infants. In that way, the dreadful potato famine could be alleviated and Ireland's surplus population reduced. It was intended to sting the British ruling class and motivate them to confront their own callous denial of Irish suffering. What really resolved the horrible famine, precipitated by the potato blight, was not British upper class largess, however, but the mass emigration of destitute Irish to American, the land of opportunity and plenty.

Why evoke Swift's "A Modest Proposal" today? The healthcare crisis that confronts the U.S. in general, and Louisiana in specific, touches 47 million Americans without health insurance. Eventually, with changes associated with the Affordable Care Act, they might be eligible for Medicaid, swelling the ranks of such recipients from the current 25% of the Louisiana population to 45% or more. This potentially amounts to two million adults and children out of Louisiana's total population of 4.5 million. This staggering number would have to be assimilated by a medical delivery system already in full-scale transformation from a state-operated public charity system into evolving "private-public partnerships." In theory, such a transformation might succeed if the resources devoted to it are commensurate with the numbers involved. That, however, remains to be seen.

Another painful reality is that the true private sector, at least in Louisiana, is not obliged to take Medicaid patients. And with the exception of Federally Qualified Health Centers (FQHCs), similar organizations and most pediatricians, the private sector shuns such individuals. Since Medicaid reimbursements, at least for outpatient services, are so low, it becomes economic suicide for most private providers to accept any significant proportion of Medicaid patients. Those that do can become swamped with such patients and either be forced to see an inordinate number of patients or change their clientele by reducing or eliminating Medicaid recipients.

Hospitals, however, cannot turn away the uninsured or underinsured (i.e. Medicaid). Due to legal mandates of the Emergency Medical Treatment and Active Labor Act (EMTALA) of 1986, they cannot turn away emergency patients unless the hospital has established the case as non-urgent. Hospitals, notably in Louisiana, used to re-direct non-paying emergency patients to the Charity system. That, however, is a practice of the past largely because of EMTALA's substantial fines and penalties associated with anything perceived as patient dumping making inappropriate transfers very onerous, indeed. In addition, the Charity system, so unique to Louisiana, and the previous destination of many uninsured and underinsured, will soon cease to exist in its former configuration, replaced by "public-private partnerships."

So what can be done? Louisiana is not doctor-poor. Although we were 48/50 for our state health outcomes in 2013 and 49/50 for our state health determinants (factors that contribute to health) in 2013, we were a respectable 20/50 for our number of primary care physicians per capita. Although physician distribution favors larger urban areas, there are enough doctors in Louisiana, at least for current demand.

What exactly is this "modest medical proposal?" Medical licensure can be tied into seeing a certain percentage of uninsured and underinsured (i.e. Medicaid) patients. At least in Louisiana, the Secretary of the Department of Health and Hospitals (DHH) could implement such a licensure requirement with the stroke of a pen. By distributing the burden of the uninsured and underinsured more equitably, that population could be successfully managed. Those physicians unwilling to comply could pay into a special fund to increase the reimbursement of those who do participate. With a DHH mandate, the underinsured and uninsured would have access to quality care throughout Louisiana.

Since our medico-legal system poses such a problem, liability would have to be offered through the State Office of Risk Management. The uninsured and underinsured are often poor and represent tempting targets for unscrupulous plaintiff's attorneys. Having the physicians assume additional medical liability for little reimbursement is clearly untenable. State insurance could act as a deterrent to lawsuits, so common in the indigent population with nothing to lose and everything to gain by litigation.

Mandating physicians to see a certain percentage of uninsured and underinsured patients, as a condition of medical licensure, is not an unrealistic or even a new proposal. Massachusetts reportedly has a similar system, which has been successfully implemented while achieving near universal health coverage. This "modest medical proposal," would, of course, generate opposition. The private sector does not want to be exposed to additional financial hardships associated with reduced reimbursement, while being exposed to increased liability. Yet what other solution exists if we want to extend quality care to all citizens?

Outpatient public-private partnerships might alleviate the need for such a drastic proposal, but the results of the current transformations will only become apparent with time. What we want to avoid is the total medical disenfranchisement of 45% of the state's population and the worsening of our already catastrophic health statistics. A concerted effort by private physicians, coupled with licensure mandates and malpractice relief, just might be the prescription for improved access to care and better health outcomes in Louisiana.

Swift, Jonathan. "A Modest Proposal for Preventing the Children of Poor People From Being a Burthen to Their Parents or Country, and for Making Them Beneficial to the Publick." S. Harding Publisher. Dublin 1729.

H. HEALTHCARE VS. WEATHCARE: AN AMERICAN DILEMMA

A curious and expensive drama has been playing out in the United State since the 1970's. Around that time, the United States and its developed partners spent about the same percentage of their Gross Domestic Products (GDPs) on healthcare. As a county's GDP rises, the percentage spent on health tends to rise, as does the per capita amount spend on health-related issues. Over the past several decades, however, a curious phenomenon occurred. The percentage (and per capita amount) spent on healthcare began increasing at an accelerated rate in the U.S. when compared with other developed countries.

Just as this took place, other countries in this group achieved universal or near-universal health coverage, while the U.S. lagged woefully behind with almost 14% of its population (or around 47 million people) uninsured. Equally disturbing were the health outcomes in the U.S. that, perhaps not coincidentally and despite massive expenditures, sank to 34th or less depending on the indicator when compared with other developed nations.

A curious and disturbing disconnect occurred between increases in life expectancy and per capital health expenditures, just as the absolute and percentage health costs skyrocketed. By 2010, health care expenditures reached 2.8 trillion dollars a years, or around 17% of the GDP (approximately three times more than defense spending). Rather than achieve "the best medical care in the world," the U.S. clearly achieved the most expensive, with mediocre outcomes in life expectancy, infant mortality, maternal mortality and other health indicators.

Why this costly disconnect? During the same time period, there has also been a steady deterioration of social capital (as defined by Robert Putnam in his book, "Bowling Alone"), with an emphasis on the individual rather than the group. There has also been an increased glorification of what Dan Beauchamp calls "market-justice" (as opposed to "social-justice.") "Market-justice" refers to an emphasis on a belief that health outcomes are related almost entirely to individual behaviors and decisions, with little or no need for collective inputs in the form of governmental regulations and policies.

The gradual rise of our own massive medico-industrial complex (what Beauchamp refers to as our "medical care complex"), accompanied by an erosion of governmental oversight, has created this perfect storm of runaway costs and stagnating results. Public health, in its broadest, sense, emphasizes the collective responsibility and also seeks to avoid the "blame the victim" philosophy so characteristic of "market-justice" proponents.

As mentioned, the U.S., alone among developed countries, has failed to achieve universal health coverage while pumping trillions of dollars annually into an insatiable medical machine. Direct-to-consumer advertising, the deregulation of so-called "dietary supplements," privatization of health care delivery, and an incredible contingency fee-driven medico-legal system have all contributed to our current healthcare disaster.

Attempts to reform the system have been met with contempt, derision and unrestrained hostility from every segment of our massive medico-industrial complex. And why not? Which part of those benefiting from the system want to see their slice of the massive pie decrease? The hospitals? The doctors? The durable medical equipment suppliers? The home health and hospice services? The pharmaceutical companies? The plaintiff attorneys? Some individuals, notably in public health, have recognized the necessity of reform, yet their voices have often been drowned out be a drumbeat of opposition from the misinformed and the cynical, many of whom benefit from the current situation.

Every system is perfectly designed to produce the outcomes it produces. Instead of insisting we have "the best medical system in the world," let us examine its shortcomings and make a good faith effort to address the problems. More market-justice will only produce more of the same unacceptable disparities. Healthcare, unlike making cars or computers, does not necessarily respond to the market. Concentrating on social-justice rather than market-justice recognizes the irrefutable evidence that developed societies with the lowest economic disparities also produce the best and most consistent health outcomes. This should be our goal and guiding principle as well.

As Martin Luther King, Jr. said "There is no health justice without social justice." For better or for worse, public health remains political at its very core. It seeks to harness collaboration between individuals and institutions in order to reduce disparities and obtain optimal health outcomes. More of our same dysfunctional system will only lead to an extension of our current expensive calamity. We cannot help but recognize, unless we refuse to see the facts or, worse yet, rationalize and embrace them, that our current system generates unequal and unacceptable results. We must ask ourselves the essential question: Do we want health for all, or just wealth for some?

Hofrichter, R., Editor. *Health and Social Justice: Politics, Ideology, and Inequity in the Distribution of Disease*, San Francisco: Jossey-Bass, A Wiley Imprint, 2003.

Putnam, R. Bowling Alone: The Collapse and Revival of American Community. New York: Simon & Schuster, 2000.

Beauchamp, D.E. "Public Health: Alien Ethic in a Strange Land?" American Journal of Public Health, 1975, 65. 1338-1339.

http://www.ncbi.nlm.nih.gov/pmc/articles/PMC1776254/

Arah, O., "On the relationship between individual and populations health," Med Health Care and Philo (2009) 12:235-244.

http://download.springer.com/static/pdf/781/art%253A10.1007%25 2Fs11019-008-9173-8.pdf?auth66=1388267345_b1a002299462c57a6 2b88640a593e996&ext=.pdf

CHAPTER X
LAGNIAPPE (A LITTLE EXTRA)

A. MEDICAL CARE IN LOUISIANA
AND THE GHOST OF HUEY P. LONG

It is said that you cannot understand the present without knowing the past and healthcare is certainly no exception. The State of Louisiana is undergoing a revolution in its healthcare delivery system, precipitated by changes at both the local and national level.

Louisiana has long suffered with a significant number of poor and unhealthy citizens. Although rich in natural resources, Louisiana has a long tradition of social and economic inequality, resulting in marked health disparities and poor health outcomes. With the discovery of huge oil deposits, companies of that time, notably Standard Oil, converged on Louisiana to extract its black gold. Governor Huey P. Long, a brilliant speaker and savvy politician, recognized the deep-seated resentments of the indigent population, made even worse by the Great Depression, as well as the opportunity to benefit from the oil bonanza.

Huey P. Long ran for governor of Louisiana on a populist platform of "Share the Wealth." He proposed that the resources that left the state must be appropriately paid for and that money should, in part, be funneled back into roads, schools, books and medical care for those unable to pay for them. This position, extremely popular with a large number of Louisiana's destitute citizens, resulted in Huey P. Long's meteoric rise to power. His populist views and organizational abilities proved an unbeatable combination. His party apparatus proliferated and he was able to establish effective control over the legislature, State Police, National Guard and civil service structure. Civil servants were obliged to forfeit a portion of their salaries for "voluntary" contributions to the Huey P. Long political machine, the famous "deduct."

One of his goals was the establishment of a world-class medical institution for the poor of Louisiana. The Charity Hospital of New Orleans was the flagship and first of a system of state-owned and state-operated medical institutions scattered throughout the state's boundaries. The Office of Public Health also expanded under the same tradition of state-delivered medical care, which continued until this decade. This heavily state-driven model is unique in the United States. Most states have county hospitals and county health departments established for the indigent. There are variable structures and functions from county to county, depending on the wealth and population. There is, however, always some state component to public health departments, but the Louisiana model is peculiar in both its regional structure and the robust state presence at the local level.

Louisiana's unique model came under critical review with changes in the political climate in the nations and in the state. The populist, state-driven system was labeled as an inefficient, expensive and archaic leftover of a bygone social era. The result has been a rapid dismantling of the state operated system and the resultant repercussions on all aspects of the health care delivery system. Since many of the medical providers grew and prospered in collaboration with the state system, a rapid and somewhat chaotic transformation has gripped Louisiana. The premise that the private sector can and will deliver better and less expensive care has driven these changes that are expected to improve both access and health outcomes.

Since Louisiana's population is still made up of over 25% Medicaid recipients and around 20% uninsured, and the state remains 48/50 in its health outcomes, caring for this mass of indigent patients remains a significant challenge. The verdict is still out as to whether this transformation in healthcare delivery can be achieved without deterioration in health outcomes. Since Louisiana has always remained close to or at the bottom in the nation for health outcomes, a further drop may not be a long ways to go, but is still undesirable. The ghost of Huey P. Long continues to haunt Louisiana, but perhaps with the dismantling of the state-driving healthcare system, that ghost will, at long last, be put to rest.

B. GIVE ME SHELTER!

Louisiana, with its extensive coastline, remains vulnerable to devastating hurricanes. No one can forget the destruction wrought by Katrina, but there has also been Rita, Gustav, Ike and Isaac to name but a few more recent storms. In response to this constant threat, Louisiana has developed a complex system of sheltering for its coastal residents. Since almost half of the state population lives near or below I-10, this becomes a huge issue.

There are, in fact, at least three types of shelters: General Shelters, Critical Transportation Needs Shelters and Medical Special Needs Shelters. General Shelters are those open to anyone driving up from South Louisiana. These are most often run by the American Red Cross, but can be opened by churches and other private organizations. Some parishes in South Louisiana make individual arrangements with parishes in Central and North Louisiana in what is called a "point to point" sheltering system.

Critical Transportation Needs Shelters (CTNS), managed by the Department of Children and Family Services (formerly Social Services), are also established in Central and North Louisiana. These are dedicated to people who do not have transportation for self-evacuation. Parish pick up points are established in key locations in South Louisiana and transportation is provided by buses, arranged in cooperation with the Department of Transportation. These evacuees are triaged (sorted) either on spot or subsequently in Baton Rouge to separate those who are medically fragile and need to go to a Medical Special Needs Shelter.

Medical Special Needs Shelters (MSNS) are manned with providers from the Office of Public Health and are also located around the state, but principally in Central and North Louisiana. The evacuees in these shelters require complex medical care and are usually accompanied by a caregiver. It is often patients who are benefiting from home health services and may include those with wound care issues, dialysis, tube feeding, oxygen therapy or other medical issues. Patients in nursing homes, hospitals and other institutions are evacuated to equivalent institutions and not into a MSNS.

Central Louisiana is blessed with a unique asset, the State Shelter at Alexandria (also known as the "Mega-Shelter.") This is a 206,000 square foot facility, located on the LSU-Ag Center property adjacent to LSU-Alexandria. It can house up to 2,500 Critical Transportation Needs evacuees and up to 450 Medical Special Needs evacuees. The logistics of operating such a facility are staggering and require the cooperation not only of the Department of Children and Family Services and the Department of Health and Hospitals (including the Office of Public Health, Behavioral Health and Medicaid), but also the Louisiana State Police, National Guard, Department of Transportation, Bureau of Emergency Medical Services and many others. Food services, laundry, waste disposal, oxygen and other necessities need to be pre-arranged by the Department of Children and Family Services.

When the Governor declares a state of emergency, a complex series of activities take place, including the formation of emergency operations centers (EOCs), organized in accordance with the National Incident Management System (NIMS). These EOCs exist at the local, regional and state levels, culminating in the Governor's Office of Homeland Security and Emergency Preparations (GOHSEP).

Louisiana, by choice and necessity, has become a leader in the development of plans for evacuation and sheltering. Central Louisiana has become not only the state's geographic hub, but also the location of Louisiana's only dedicated sheltering facility. We have long been known for our hospitality and now we are also known for our sheltering capacity. Even though there is an extensive state system, every individual still needs to have their own evacuation and sheltering plans. With all of its resources, the state still cannot shelter each and every individual. While there is a collective obligation, there must also be a personal responsibility. Since disasters can strike anywhere, anytime, have a plan!

www.getagameplan.org

C. COMMUNITY HEALTH WORX:
HELPING TO FILL THE MEDICAL VOID

Louisiana, like much of the United States, has a serious problem of uninsured or underinsured citizens. Over 20% of Louisianans have no insurance at all and about 25% benefit from Medicaid. For the latter, the problem is more related to the paucity of Medicaid providers than not having insurance per se. Having a Medicaid card does not necessarily equate to having access to health care, but it is better than having no insurance at all.

Since the cost of insurance mirrors that of medical care, the steady increase in costs, particularly in the United States, has priced many Americans out of the insurance market. Because unmet medical needs has been an on-going problem throughout Louisiana and the nation, a network of institutions has been developed to address that segment of the population that makes too much money to qualify for Medicaid, but not enough to purchase health insurance.

To address this large and growing number of citizens, Dr. C.D. Lowrey, then Medical Director of Rapides Regional Medical Center, put together the project of a "free" clinic for the working poor. Incorporated on February 15, 1999, the Working People's Free Clinic opened its doors and began seeing patients. Linda Holinga was hired as the first and remains the current Executive Director. In 2005, the Caring People's Free Pharmacy was incorporated with the Free Clinic into a new entity, "Community Health Worx."

Patients who cannot afford health insurance and meet the financial eligibility of 200% of the federal poverty level and who do not qualify for Medicaid or other insurance will be seen in the clinic at no charge. Every Tuesday and Thursday, volunteer physicians, nurse practitioners and nurses work with other non-medical staff (both volunteer and paid) to process and see patients. Medications are provided through the pharmacy, which works with volunteers to do the voluminous paperwork associated with pharmaceutical firms' patient assistance programs. Those medications not available through donations or patient assistance plans are purchased with the operating funds.

Prescriptions are also provided on a "one time fill" basis to persons with valid prescriptions, who are encouraged to see if they meet eligibility for more long-term services.

At least 1000 active patients use Community Health Worx as their medical home. Over 3,000 have been served in that capacity over the years. Some will eventually find jobs with associated health insurance or others will become eligible for Medicaid or Medicare or other insurance plans through the Affordable Care Act. While waiting, however, Community Health Worx helps bridge the gap. In November 2011, in collaboration with area dentists and the local dental society, a dental clinic began which sees patients on Thursday nights. Although it is an "extraction only" dental clinic, it helps keep patients from the revolving door of emergency services.

Agreements with both Rapides Regional Medical Center and CHRISTUS-St. Frances Cabrini Hospital help provide laboratory and x-ray services. Other medical groups provide occasional services, including pathology, biopsies and some specific radiological procedures. Community Health Worx collaborates with LSU-HSC-Huey P. Long and LSU-Shreveport for some referral services. Despite these intense collaborations, the unmet medical need is steadily increasing.

Although medical-legal protection is offered to volunteering physicians and other professional through special legislation, it is still difficult to recruit adequate providers. Of the over 300 local physicians in the Alexandria-Pineville area, only a handful of dedicated souls give consistently of their time and talents. They, like all the other dental and non-medical volunteers, deserve the community's thanks and admiration. If you cannot give of your time, Community Health Worx appreciates your donations. Charity should begin at home, and our medically needy are no exception. Please call 318-767-9979 if you are interested in donating either your services or money.

D. DELTA CARE PROJECT: INNOVATIVE READINESS TRAINING IN FERRIDAY, LOUISIANA

The equipment has been shipped away and the soldiers have flown off to their respective homes around the United States (many from the Northeast) after a successful Innovative Readiness Training, which took place in Ferriday, Louisiana, from August 8-16, 2013.

The project, the brainchild of Mrs. Vicki Riser (Delta Regional Network) and Mrs. Heather Malone (Concordia Economic and Industrial Development), started with a grant request to the U.S. Army to come to Ferriday, Louisiana as a location for an Innovative Readiness Training. These trainings, destined for Army Reservists, are intended to bring medical, dental, optometric (glasses) and veterinary services to areas of need within the United States. By targeting areas of medical need, the Army Reservists can bring much needed services to areas within the borders of the U.S. and also train for deployments elsewhere in the world.

When the U.S. Army accepted the grant request in January 2013, there began an intense and prolonged period of meetings and preparations for the event. Several teams from the U.S. Army (fulltime and reservists) came down to Ferriday to reconnoiter and coordinate with the civilian authorities, notably Mrs. Riser and Mrs. Malone. They came to confirm the services, location, availability of local resources and other logistic considerations. Eventually, weekly phone conferences helped work out details of the project, now named the Delta Care Project, which took place in the Central Louisiana Technical Community College at Ferriday. The Community College proved the perfect venue for such a project and both the site and personnel performed admirably. Other local sites were established for veterinary services and the making of eyeglasses.

Despite some last minute issues related to credentialing (a complex issue when personnel under military orders work outside of a military facility within U.S. borders), doors opened as planned on August 8,

2013. Because of intense pre-event publicity, coordinated through local civilian authorities including the Office of Public Health, there was a terrific local and regional response to the event. A combination of appointments and walk-ins received medical, dental and optometric services over the course of the following 9 days. Local volunteers helped with the appointments and many other aspects of patient processing.

Over 3,600 grateful residents from all over East Central Louisiana and West Central Mississippi received quality care. Patients underwent over 1000 dental procedures and over 900 glasses were created on site. Over 500 medical patients were seen, many of whom had hypertension and diabetes, sometimes previously diagnosed and sometimes not. Around 80 animals received veterinary services (including spaying and neutering) in cooperation with the Adams County Humane Society in Mississippi.

In short, this was a win-win situation for the citizens of Louisiana and the U.S. Army Reserve. The former received care and the latter received training. Major Compliment and his team held a VIP Press Conference on August 9, 2013, attended by local elected officials, state officials, and U.S. Army representatives from Washington. The closing ceremony, including presentation of Certificates of Appreciation for U.S. Army Reserve team members and local authorities, took place on August 17, 2013. As an example of successful military-civilian operations, it may well serve as a model of other such initiatives in other parts of Louisiana and other states.

E. MEDICAL MALPRACTICE:
THE MOST INSIDIOUS CANCER

The medico-legal climate in the United States defies reason. It is, of course, tied into a whole approach to liability that is, alas, typically American. Although some may cringe when other national solutions are suggested, it is useful to see how other societies handle the universal problem of malpractice. The Belgian model deserves consideration.

First, contingency fees are illegal in Belgium. There is no such thing as a lawyer taking a percentage of a potential award. Legal fees may be high, but they are hourly fees, much as you would expect from a skilled mechanic or electrician. By removing the motivation of enormous economic windfalls to lawyers, the number of lawsuits drops dramatically. The price of malpractice insurance also drops accordingly (ten times less in Belgium than in the United States). Removing the insidious practice of contingency fees would remove a good part of the profit incentive that drives the current American malpractice and other personal injury industry.

Lawyers argue that eliminating contingency fees would deny legal access to the poor. Not so! The issue here is not justice, but greed. And the corrosive effect of unbridled greed poisons the practice of law, just as it can poison medicine and any other aspects of our society.

Second, malpractice cases in Belgium are handled by judges specialized in the field of medical malpractice, and not before juries. As noble and as intelligent as the general population may be, the tremendous complexities of modern medicine and the passions whipped up in the jury system in such cases, makes trial by jury more of a liability than an asset. Using specialized judges, instead of juries, removes the element of public passion, so unhelpful in complex medical cases.

Third, specialized malpractice judges in Belgium are appointed for their expertise, and not elected. Although this does not completely remove the politics from the system, it greatly reduces the political and monetary pressures exerted by attorneys on judges. Appointing judges removes or at least reduces the politics in the process.

Profit, passion and politics all work together to make our medico-legal system an unmitigated disaster, a true cancer in our society. The threat of malpractice and the omnipresent tendency to "cover your ass," has gradually infiltrated the process of medical care. Instead of assuming responsibility for the patient until their problems exceed your level of competence, every specialist needs to be consulted, not so much for the benefit they bring to the patient's care, but for the protection their opinion offers in case of litigation. Another sad result of the current atmosphere is that every patient is transformed from a trusted partner in the doctor-patient relationship to a potential litigant to be feared. In no way does this enhance patient care. On the contrary, it results in a progressive erosion of trust and a total corruption of the patient-doctor relationships, plus a proliferation of questionable and expensive tests and consultations. That increases medical costs in a system that is already twice as expensive per person as any other medical system in most other countries of the developed world, and with less than favorable outcomes.

The problems of health care are universal. Every country has its burden of heart disease, cancer, infectious diseases, and other health problems. But medico-legal systems, much like healthcare delivery systems, are manmade. Let us choose wisely when we embark on the challenge of changing our healthcare delivery system. We cannot neglect elements, such as tort reform, that we must address in order to make our system one of the best and most financially sustainable in the world, not just the most expensive.

F. ON BEING SUED: AN OPEN LETTER TO MY YOUNGER COLLEAGUES

"When the heart is full, it spills out of the mouth."
An African proverb

As someone engaged in pursuing a medical career, you have embarked on an extraordinary journey to become one of mankind's most honored professionals, a doctor. Although there seems to be an unlimited supply of lawyer jokes, how many doctor jokes have your heard lately? Doctors are, indeed, maligned for greed and arrogance, but those criticisms remain directed toward an abstract group. Patients almost invariably say that they distrust doctors in general, but not their personal physician in whom they place their total confidence. From a physician's standpoint, you may condemn or vilify the attitudes of the general public, while maintaining an equally trusted bond with your personal patients.

Mutual trust must exist in order to maintain that mysterious entity we call the patient-physician relationship. It inspires physicians to work long hours, sacrifice family activities, curtail personal interests and stay up at night to deal with emergencies. Do physicians earn money for their services? Of course they do, and often amounts that largely exceed average national incomes. Yet the desire to make money cannot, in the long run, sustain a physician's motivation to continue in his or her profession.

Physicians must struggle to be admitted to medical school, struggle to complete training, struggle to fulfill their duties as physicians, and struggle to maintain a level of professional competence, including professional re-certification. Overshadowing these struggles, the specter of litigation looms like an unwanted medical complication.

Sooner or later, through mischance or mistake, most physicians will be sued. The process lasts years and the results are devastating. Regardless of the merits of the case, which can range from the well deserved to those without medical merit (so-called frivolous suits), the process turns into an intense psychological marathon for the doctor.

Once sued, a string of legal maneuvers begin, including requests for records, meetings with your attorney, depositions by you and other concerned parties including the patient, expert witnesses and others. This dreary and prolonged process may end up in the courtroom.

The plaintiff's attorney contends, of course, that you are a bad doctor. Your errors, real or imagined, may include poor records, omissions, failure to diagnose and treat, or even willful misconduct, all of which allegedly violate the national standard of medical care. You will have the dubious privilege of hearing qualified expert witnesses denounce your actions as inadequate or even dangerous and resulting in a cascade of errors leading to the patient's harm or death. This, of course, despite having done the best you could under difficult circumstances.

Some of you may even choose to practice in challenging places, where disease, poverty, and the lack of medical resources limit access to care. To those who have chosen to practice in areas of medical need, the distress of litigation will seem all the more egregious and painful. You will feel an extraordinary sense of betrayal, not from the legal community, from whom vicious attacks should be expected, but from your own community of academic colleagues. You will ask yourselves how you could undergo the tribulations of practice, especially in rural or depressed urban areas, and be held to national standards of care developed and propagated from distant urban academic centers. Indeed, we are one nation, and universal standards of care, while justified in the abstract, are hardly possible in our complex reality. Yet the discordance between the reality and the expectations remains the medico-legal norm.

If you believe that your learned colleagues in academic institutions will help to reconcile this difference and admire you for your efforts, do not be deceived. The zeal with which supposedly honored and trusted colleagues attack and discredit you will make your head spin and your heart sink. We have all looked to the ivory tower of academia for continued education and help with referrals in complex cases. But among academicians are those that have lost touch with their role as mentors and educators and assumed the role of persecutors. Our medico-legal system, as irrational and self-serving as it is, can reach into the ivory tower and find those individuals only too willing to sell their opinions and thus become part of the problem rather than part of the solution of caring for the health of our citizens.

Just as that element of trust must exist between physicians and patients, it must also exist between physicians and their consultants, especially those in the academic world. Even for those among us with the most hardened psyches, it comes as a shock to see colleagues in academic medicine, those who we view as leaders and mentors, choose to attack us with joyful enthusiasm. They would not dare to treat their immediate colleagues or referring physicians with such perfidy, but some anonymous fool from a distant state can be treated with supposed impunity. No such impunity exists, however. Once our learned colleagues have cashed their checks and returned to their daily routine, the corrosive effect of this lack of solidity will gnaw at their moral fiber until little sense of collegiality remains, if it ever existed at all.

And what is the profession of medicine without collegiality? Is it a constant warfare between the weak and the powerful, a battle to the death for economic supremacy? And in this insidious mêlée, what becomes of the patient? And is the doctor who betrays his colleague's trust, the same doctor revered by his patients for both his competence and compassion, still worthy of their respect and confidence? Can and should we separate our morality between the courtroom and the examining room?

When we ridicule and debase our colleagues instead of educating and nurturing them, we have lost all sense of morality. Do we have the right to wear a white coat if we have the blackest of souls? Of course we do, since hypocrisy knows no bounds. But the insidious nature of hypocrisy contaminates the soul, just as it does the entire edifice of medicine, and continues to do so until both may collapse from the ensuing rot.

Those of you who work in rural and semi-rural areas without adequate medical resources will be required to refer patients out of town. Any of you with some years of experience will recognize that you can get helpful responses from out-of-town specialists. You sometimes, however, receive only a written consultation, while your patient never returns to you. Or, worse yet, the big city consultant may accuse you of having made an erroneous or delayed diagnosis and treatment, thus setting the stage for future litigation.

Once the poison of mistrust has entered into the patient's mind, instilled by the thoughtless or unscrupulous remarks of the consultant, the physician-patient relationship with the primary care physician can wither and die, if not be killed outright. Why does this happen? Most consultants try and perform a creditable service to their referring physicians and they are, in fact, our honored and trusted colleagues. Some, however, cannot resist the temptation to aggrandize themselves at the expense of their hapless referring physicians.

Into this mix of hidden dangers, the legal system encourages litigation through the ubiquitous practice of contingency fees (receiving 40% or more of an eventual settlement or award). This profit driven system, which infects our society as a whole, also results in a proliferation of professional expert witnesses, each one willing and able to denounce their colleagues.

The end result for the practicing physician is that, if you have a large active practice, you will find yourself defending your competence against those whose sole motivation is to discredit you. You might say that you are willing and able to confront this menace. Yet, as everyone knows, we could always have done better: better documentation, better follow-up, and better patient education. And since no one is perfect, there is always a possibility for criticism, even when the care is excellent.

So what are the solutions? Broad ranging medico-legal reforms, while desirable, are unlikely. The current system creates an army of people with vested interests in the present system. Doctors, just like lawyers or expert witnesses, are all part of our 2.8 trillion dollar a year medico-legal industry, which shows little signs of slowing down.

When you are sued, take heart that you are not the only one who has suffered. Your patient, by definition, has also undergone a tort, an injury of some sort, whether real or imagined and perhaps not even related to your care. Once you have received the fateful papers with your name vs. that former (or sometimes incredibly enough a current patient), you are off for a multi-year extravaganza. You will turn over every aspect of the case in your mind, see it from every angle you can imagine, and ride a rollercoaster of emotions from anger to denial to depression, not unlike someone given the diagnosis of cancer. Since life goes on, you will put the case in the back of your mind. But when you have finally more or less forgotten the case, it will return with a vengeance, triggered by any numbers of events: a request for additional information, or a deposition by one of the actors in this drama, or some random correspondence from your attorney. You will plunge again into endless days and nights of painful introspection and soul searching. Ultimately, you will hear the patient, joined by expert witnesses, engage in an orgy of criticism of your best, good faith efforts to help them.

Worst of all, when you want to discuss the horror and indignity of your experience, you will be instructed by your own counsel not to discuss the case with anyone, especially your medical colleagues. This flies in the face of everything you tell your own patients about discussing their problems with friends, family, clergy or counseling professionals. With your patients, you stress the therapeutic value of communication as opposed to the malignant effects of isolation. Yet you will be told not to discuss your case with anyone, especially your professional colleagues.

At this point, the temptation may be to throw money at the problem so it will go away. You may lean toward a settlement, if only to have some peace of mind. Do not be tempted! As painful and difficult as it may appear, it is better to be judged before a jury (even if they are not your peers) than to give money in the vain attempt to make the problem go away. Driven by greed, the complexity of medicine, and a wave of unrealistic expectations from the public, this problem of litigation and its poisonous effect on medicine will not be resolved, at least not at this time and especially not by paying off the plaintiff's attorney. Whether you settle or lose in court, you will still be put in the national database for every insurance company and hospital credentialing committee to ponder over and pick to pieces.

My heart goes out to each and every one of you, my young colleagues. Look deep into the sources of your personal strength, wherever it may come from, and remember that the vast majority of your patients believe in you, despite your imperfections and frailties. They hold you to standards of humanity, not perfection, and you should do the same for them. When and if you reach the point that your mistrust has infected your relationships with all of your patients, who you now regard as potential litigants, you may have to leave the beloved profession that you have struggled so hard to achieve. Your departure, as tragic as it may be for your patients and the community, will be a small price to pay for your personal sanity.

Should you choose to stay and fight for your patients, your practice, your privilege to care for the sick and the distressed, how can you achieve it? The paradox lies in being able to desensitize yourself to the medico-legal process. You must arm yourself with a carapace of indifference to assaults from colleagues, especially academicians, and plaintiff's attorneys who seek to benefit from the miseries that inevitable come from dealing with sickness and death.

Yet at what price comes this carapace of indifference? The very quality that makes us good physicians is that ability to empathize. It is that inherent sensitivity to the conditions of our patients that makes us good doctors, yet also paradoxically places us in a position of extreme vulnerability. Who can turn their sensitivity on and off without losing their very soul, their capacity to be humane? And isn't that what medicine is all about, being humane?

So do not sacrifice those qualities that make you a good doctor in every sense of the word. We all know that technical proficiency and material success do not make a doctor good without that accompanying ability to feel deeply and sincerely for the patient. And if you lose this quality, you lose the very soul of medicine.

Be strong and be good, regardless of how you are treated by your colleagues, who sometimes merit neither honor nor trust. As mentioned above, when the empathy in you dies and the cost of performing medicine becomes a poisonous effort, take the path you must even if it means abandoning the profession you have struggled so hard to attain.

*"And if you cannot work with love but only with distaste, it
is better that you should leave your work and sit at the gate
of the temple and take alms of those who work with joy."*
Khalil Gibran

If this misfortune should befall you, be prepared to suffer the loss
of those many relationships with good and decent people, whose
consideration and respect buoy up your daily life. Be prepared to
pass through a looking glass away from the high-pressure world of
drug reps and home health representatives, salesmen and hospital
administrators, who barely mask their naked self-interest. Other doors
can and will open and despite everything, you will remain a doctor, a
profession still respected by most. There will still be the sick to heal,
although perhaps outside of the traditional venues of medicine. There
will even be those precious locations where you can practice for free
without the sinister specter of litigation. You will find those who
still require our expertise and who have fallen outside of the dubious
protection of our established medical system: the poor, the uninsured,
the unemployed and mentally unstable.

Your sensitivity, your very soul as a physician and a person are a stake
in the daily choices you make, and that is why this awful internal
struggle is so important. You can be on the side of greed and evil or,
if you can take the crushing responsibility, continue your lofty work
until the drudgery exceeds the joy and empathy evaporates from your
soul, leaving it as parched and sterile as a lunar landscape.

If, or rather when, you must end up in court, take courage. Perhaps
in a jury you may find those people who have retained a shred of
humanity and the intelligence to understand complex medical
concepts. Although you swoon before the effort, you will have to
educate twelve random men and women about complicated and
controversial medical issues. Do not be afraid to confront the
nightmare of a trial, as imperfect and illogical as the system appears.
To not do so is to capitulate in the face naked aggression.

Capitulation will not lead to change either in you or in our insane
medico-legal system. If you must drink the awful brew of litigation,
then drink it down to the last poisonous drop in the hope that some

good may yet come from the process. Live and work in the hope that our pernicious system may yet undergo reform, as unlikely as that now appears. And remember that each day and with each action, we have the choice of being part of the solution or part of the problem.

Take the high road, however painful, wherever it may lead. Therein lays your salvation as an individual and any hope that we might yet create a better world for everyone. And what other goal is there for a person, especially a physician?

G. SOCIAL CAPITAL
AND HEALTH OUTCOMES

In 2000, Robert Putnam published his analysis of America's social disintegration in "Bowling Alone in America." He developed the notion of "social capital," a measure of those factors and behaviors that tend to glue societies together. Various elements go into quantifying "social capital", including his five categories: measures of community organizations, measures of personal engagement in public life, measures of volunteerism, measures of informal sociability and measures of trust. Within these categories are subgroups including things such as the number of 501(c)3's (tax exempt organizations), voting participation, membership in civic organizations, the frequency with which we invite friends over for dinner parties, whether we think most people can be trusted, and a variety of other indices of sociability and social engagement.

The South in general and Louisiana in particular, may appear to be very sociable. After all, we have a plethora of groups and organizations, from Mardi Gras Krewes to garden clubs. But when compared with other states, our level of social capital is very low. In fact, we found ourselves at the bottom of the list, along with our usual Southern neighbors, Mississippi, Alabama and Arkansas. Why should we care? And what does this have to do with public health?

It turns out that the level of social capital is directly (or indirectly) proportional to a number of health factors. Low social capital corresponds with higher rates of child poverty, higher adult incarceration, and higher number of hours of television watched by children. Low social capital also corresponds to lower high school and college graduation rates, and lower indices for overall health factors.

Why is this important? It is important because our problems of public health are not isolated from the general level of social capital in the society. It is not about one particular health factor or social issue, but a whole approach to social engagement and social cohesion. When we join a club, participate in a meeting, have friends over for dinner, or vote in elections, we are helping to enhance the social capital in our communities, our state and our nation. Mr. Putnam has made a distinction between what he called "bonding social capital" and "bridging social capital." The former (bonding) brings together people with similar backgrounds, races, incomes, religions or other social traits. It is important, but not as important for social capital as "bridging social capital," which brings together those who do not share the same social or physical attributes. Organizations that enhance bridging social capital enhance the cohesiveness of the whole society rather than simply elements within it.

As we withdraw into the cocoon of more and more restricted social activity, this impacts not only our personal health, but that of the entire community. States with high social capital are healthier states. Conversely, states with low social capital are unhealthier. As citizens, we need to seek to enhance those groups and organizations that increase the bridging social capital and thus bring together as diverse elements as possible.

Everyone should be cognizant of their personal health, whether it concerns weight control, blood pressure control, cholesterol level or cancer screening. That, however, is not sufficient. A healthy individual needs to be part of a healthy community. The individual, just like his family, his neighborhood, or his church, should be part of an every expanding series of concentric units that interact and interlock, creating the sturdy fabric of a healthy society. We need to progress from isolated elements to bonding and ultimately to bridging with those around us, the more diverse, the better. Increased social capital will inevitably result with its byproduct of increased individual and collective health.

Putnam, Robert D., "Bowling Alone, the Collapse and Revival of American Society," Simon and Schuster Paperbacks, NY, 2000.

www.americashealthrankings.org

H. CAPITAL SOCIAL ET RESULTATS DE SANTE EN LOUISIANE

En l'an 2000, Monsieur Robert Putnam a publié "Bowling Alone in America. The Collapse and Revival of American Community." Dans ce livre, il introduit l'idée du capital social ("social capital"). Il définit l'index de capital social avec cinq paramètres : les mesures d'organisation communautaire, les mesures d'engagement personnel dans la vie publique, les mesures de volontarisme, les mesures de sociabilité informelle et les mesures de confiance sociale. Tous ces paramètres tentent de mesurer la cohésion communautaire et n'ont rien à faire à première vue avec la santé publique.

Putnam a mesuré ces cinq paramètres dans chaque état des Etats-Unis et il a trouvé que les états du sud ont tous des valeurs très basses, en particulier la Géorgie, l'Alabama, le Mississippi, le Tennessee et la Louisiane. Cette distinction était aussi partagée par le Nevada, un état en croissance rapide et désorganisée socialement, contrastant avec des états du sud traditionnels. Ceux-ci partagent, non seulement des valeurs très basses de capital social, mais aussi une histoire lourde d'esclavagisme et d'inégalité sociale, perpétuée par la ségrégation légale jusqu'aux années soixante. La Louisiane, comme le Mississippi, l'Alabama et la Géorgie ont aussi un pourcentage plus élevé de population noire, comparé aux autres états des Etats-Unis.

Monsieur Putnam ne s'est pas contenté de mesurer le capital social, il a voulu aussi explorer la possibilité de corrélations entre l'index de capital social et d'autres paramètres. Ces résultats étaient aussi fascinant que troublant. Bien que ces mesures de capital social n'aient rien à voir à première vue avec d'autres paramètres de santé ou de criminalité, il a démontré qu'il y avait une corrélation étroite entre l'index de capital social et certains aspects sociaux.

Notamment, il y a une corrélation directe entre le capital social d'un état et les mesures de bien-être social. Quand le capital social d'un état est élevé, les résultats de santé publique, le bien-être des enfants, la tolérance sociale, l'égalité économique et sociale et les résultats scolaires sont meilleurs. Par contre, quand le capital social est très bas, il y a des taux élevés de meurtres, d'intolérance, d'inégalité économique et sociale, et même une augmentation dans les heures de télévisions que les enfants regardent par jour.

Les résultats de Putnam datent des années nonante, mais on peut vérifier facilement la véracité et la continuité de ces trouvailles avec les données actuelles. La "United Health Foundation" publie chaque année « America's Health Rankings » (www.americashealthrankings.org). La Louisiane continue à être le 49ième état sur 50 dans les paramètres de mesures de santé. Elle est aussi 45ième ou plus bas pour les valeurs de maladies chroniques, de mortalité infantile, de personnes sans assurances de santé, d'hospitalisations évitables, de maladies infectieuses (y compris les maladies à transmission sexuelle), et d'autres paramètres également néfastes. « Kid's Count » (www.kidscount.org) place la Louisiane 49ième sur 50 pour la condition générale des enfants. Cet état a aussi le taux le plus élevé de meurtres aux E.U. ainsi que le taux le plus élevé d'adultes incarcérés : plus de 800 pour 100,000 habitants, ce qui est le double du taux national et huit fois celui de l'Europe. Trois quarts des prisonniers en Louisiane sont noirs (les noirs représentent 33 pourcents de la population de l'état). Ces données sont similaires pour le Mississippi et l'Alabama.

A première vue, la participation dans les organisations sociales locales, le nombre de fois que l'on reçoit des amis chez soi, ou le taux de volontarisme (tous éléments de l'index de capital social) ne semblent pas avoir une corrélation directe sur la scolarité, la santé, le bien-être social ou l'égalité entre les races, et pourtant, tous ces faits sont liés entre eux.

Malgré ce déluge de mauvaises nouvelles, notamment pour la Louisiane, il y a aussi de l'espoir. Investir plus d'argent dans l'infrastructure au niveau de l'état n'est pas suffisant pour améliorer les données, il faut aussi un changement dans l'état d'esprit du public général. Une participation active dans la vie civique est directement liée à une amélioration de la santé publique. Bien sûr, il faut des infirmières, des médecins, des cliniques et des écoles pour contribuer à la santé et à la scolarité, mais il faut aussi un esprit de solidarité sociale et civique.

M. Putnam a non seulement développé l'idée du capital social, il a aussi fait une distinction entre le « bonding social capital » et le

« bridging social capital. » « Bonding social capital » est représenté dans les associations entres les gens qui partagent les mêmes intérêts, les mêmes revenus, la même race ou la même religion. Les églises, si nombreuses aux Etats-Unis, en sont des exemples. « Bridging social capital » par contre, est représenté dans les associations entres les gens qui ne partagent pas les mêmes origines sociales, ni les mêmes revenus, ni la même langue ou religion (le « Boys and Girls Club », par exemple). C'est parmi les associations de ce type que M. Putnam trouve le plus grand espoir d'augmentation du capital social. Notre obligation en tant qu'individus est de trouver et de favoriser les initiatives qui cultivent le « bridging social capital ». Celles-ci auront une influence positive indéniable sur l'index social et en conséquence sur la santé publique.

Références:

Putnam, Robert D., « Bowling Alone. The Collapse and Revival of American Community, (Simon and Schuster Paperbacks, New York, 2000.)

www.americashealthrankings.org

www.kidscount.org

ABOUT THE AUTHOR

Dr. David J. Holcombe was born in San Francisco, California in 1949 and was raised in the East Bay Area in the shadow of Mount Diablo (in Contra Costa County). He received a B.S.A. from the University of California at Davis in 1971 and a M.S.A. from the Institute of Food and Agricultural Sciences at the University of Florida in Gainesville in 1975. He subsequently traveled to Belgium for medical school, where he graduated with an M.D. from the Catholic University of Louvain in Brussels in 1981. He completed a residency in internal medicine at a Johns-Hopkins affiliated clinic in Baltimore in 1986. He and his wife and children moved to Alexandria, Louisiana, where he worked as an internist at a multi-specialty clinic for the next 20 years. In 2007, he changed his orientation and began to work in public health in Central Louisiana.

During his academic training and subsequent professional career, Dr. Holcombe has continued to write, paint and folk dance. His self-published works include collections of short stories, "Like Honored and Trusted Colleagues" and "Cappuccino at Podgorica," and short plays, "Beauty and the Botox" and "Old South, New South, No South." Since 2004, eight of his plays have been produced at the Spectral Sisters Productions annual Ten Minute Play Festival in Alexandria, Louisiana. He and his charming wife, Nicole, continue to live in Alexandria, where they contribute to the cultural life of the city, region and state. Dr. Holcombe regularly submits medical articles to various local publications, many of which appear in this volume, "Mendel's Garden: Selected Medical Topics." He serves on many advisory committees and boards, and serves as the volunteer Medical Director for Community Health Worx, a local working people's free clinic, and a volunteer Civil Surgeon for the Interfaith Immigration Group of Central Louisiana.

"MENDEL'S GARDEN: SELECTED MEDICAL TOPICS" contains a collection of short non-fiction texts covering a wide variety of medical issues. Dr. Holcombe intends each short text for the lay audience, and there are consequently no rigorous references as would be found in scientific publications. Instead, the topics are intended to introduce the average reader to a number of current issues that affect the public, from cancer to *Cyclospora* and from contingency fees to health care costs. While understanding that medical publication are out of date before they are published, there should still be something of interest for just about everyone. Feel free to hop from subject to subject and share them with friends and colleagues. Medicine should be accessible to everyone in all of its good, bad and ugly aspects.

Cover design: "Cranial Inspiration: Portrait of Dr. David Holcombe," by Terry Strickland.